HEAR BETTER, LIVE BETTER

Advice From The EarNerd

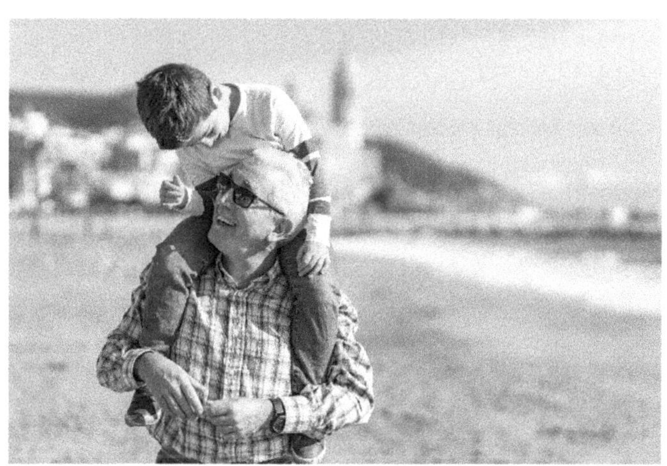

Jewell Baggett-Strehlau, Au.D.

TABLE OF CONTENTS

HEAR BETTER, LIVE BETTER

Advice From The EarNerd

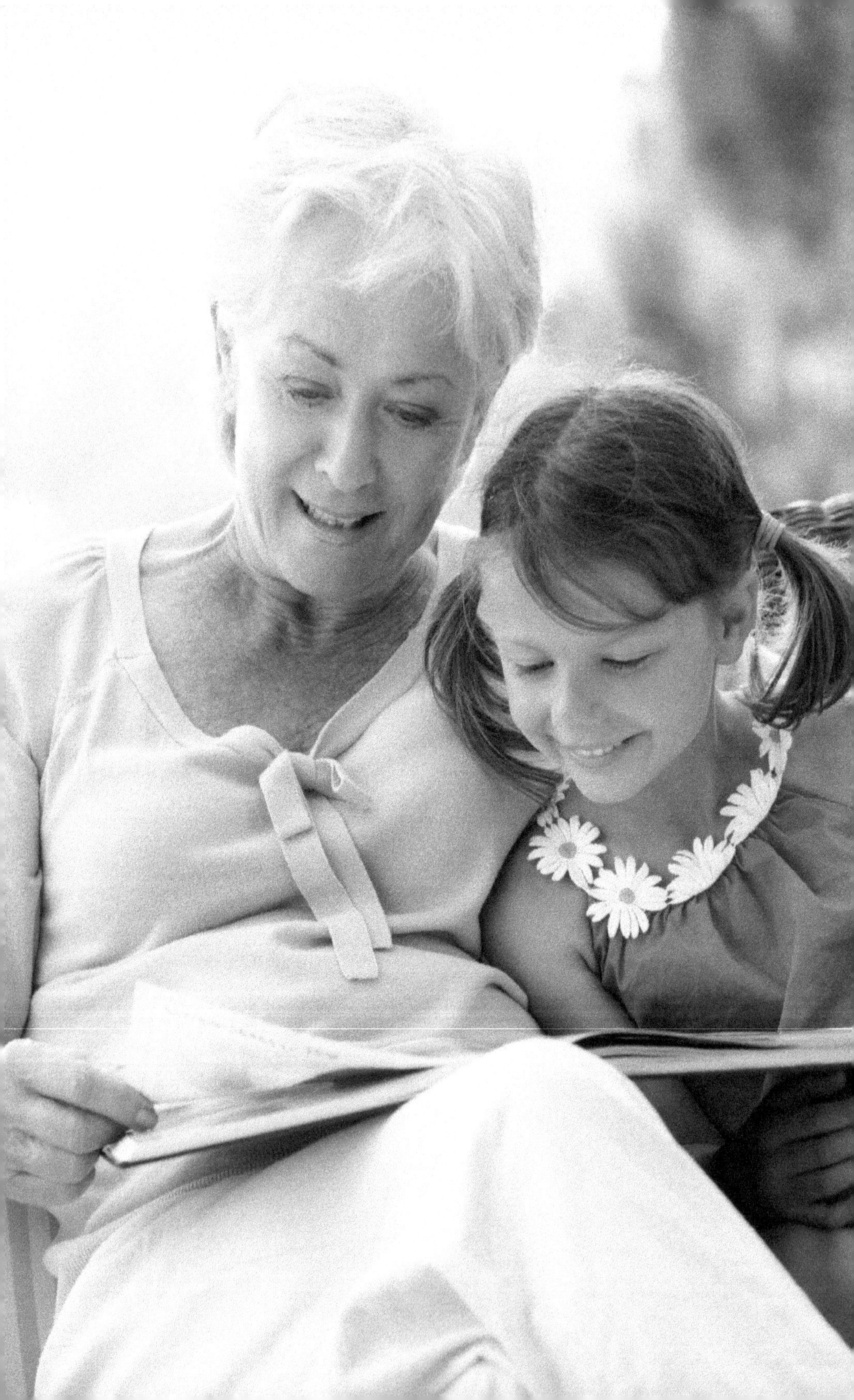

PREFACE

TODAY, APPROXIMATELY 48 MILLION PEOPLE in the United States are suffering from hearing loss. Yet nearly 40 million of them go without treatment. Many people do not understand the implications of hearing loss, which is why I wrote this book.

- *Do you want to remain independent and live an active life as you age?*
- *Did you know that hearing problems, even at the mildest stage, can lead to social isolation and increase the risk of dementia?*
- *Do you or a loved one have impaired hearing?*

Hi, I'm Dr. Jewell Baggett-Strehlau, Au.D., aka the "EarNerd" and a practicing clinical audiologist. Since my last name is one of those long, hyphenated ones and not the best for those with hearing loss, I ask my patients to call me Dr. Jewell. It's a lot easier to remember, so that is how I will be referred to in this book.

If you or a loved one has answered yes to any of the above questions, I encourage you to read this book and learn how you can live a better, more active, more engaged, and healthier life as you age. For almost 40 years, I have been helping my patients and their loved ones break free of their hearing loss and live active, engaged lives—free of the worry, stress, and medical consequences of untreated hearing loss.

Hearing is what connects us to others, to our lives and our loved ones. Hearing is a requirement for every personal and professional relationship we have; it is the building block of communication.

Hearing is also one of the major senses; in fact, I believe it is the single most important sense we have. Hearing plays a major role in our fight or flight, prey vs. predator, and history as human beings, and hearing today has the important role of keeping us communicating and connected with the world around us—at home, at work, and in our community. To further support my claim that hearing is the single most important sense we have, I offer the fact that the organ of hearing, the cochlea (aka the inner ear), is embedded deeply in the skull, in the hardest bone in our entire body, the temporal bone, giving our organ of hearing the highest level of protection.

I have put together this book to help you understand the dire consequences of untreated hearing loss and to introduce you to how today's medical options for treating hearing loss can not only help improve hearing, but also improve cognitive function, decrease your risk of developing dementia, depression, and falling, while also increasing your physical activity, and helping you live a happier and healthier lifestyle as you actively age.

Hearing loss has been listed by the Department of Health and Human Services as the third most common chronic health condition affecting seniors. Third! Hearing loss is estimated to affect nearly 50% of adults between the age of sixty to seventy years young, nearly 67% of adults between seventy to eighty years young, and the numbers only go up from there. As we live longer and science continues to increase life expectancy, we need to be best prepared to deal with this debilitating disorder and understand how it can impact our lives.

My journey up to this point has been filled with almost forty years of experience—from student to clinician in an ENT office, to working in the public school system, to hearing aid design with a major hearing aid manufacturer, to where I am now in private practice as a provider and daily patient advocate. I was lucky to discover what I love to do early in life, and as a result I have the good fortune to work with patients and their families every day as they embark on the journey of improved hearing and clarity.

I always knew I wanted to work in the sciences. I was fascinated by biology (even when dissecting a frog back in high school!) I also loved music, having sung in children's choirs since age 5, and being taught piano by my fabulously talented grandmother (she was of a generation where few women had college degrees, but she had one in music).

In college, while perusing the course catalog (remember those?), I found Speech Pathology and Audiology. It had LOTS of biology but not a lot of math, which appealed to me. The first day of my "Introduction to Audiology" class, taught by Dr. Perry completely hooked me. It combined my love of biology to my love of music and sound. The EarNerd was born!

By the way, I found out later, that audiology uses a whole lot of math. (Sigh) I found my purpose in life: to figure out what is going on with a person's hearing, how to help them understand their issues with their hearing, and to improve the process of communication in their daily lives, and it has been a marvelous experience.

Another area of interest for me has always been how the brain works. I've had long discussions with neurologist friends about brain function and concentrated much of my independent continuing education in that area of study. As a doctor of audiology with years of experience in helping people hear better, I have a unique perspective on how the brain works with sound and how hearing relates to overall health, well-being, and cognitive function. I also understand how treating hearing loss early (even before it becomes a problem that you and everybody around you can notice) significantly impacts your overall health and cognitive function and how it may significantly reduce your risk of developing dementia.

I know that I am blessed to have the capability of transforming lives and families every single day. Treating hearing loss is not magic. It is the perfect mix of science, experience, and the art of listening to people, which allows myself and my team to use advances in medical treatment of hearing loss, NeuroTechnology™ to stimulate the brain, improve cognitive function and mental health, and help adults remain independent. And the best part—it is simple for patients to manage and it's more affordable than most people think.

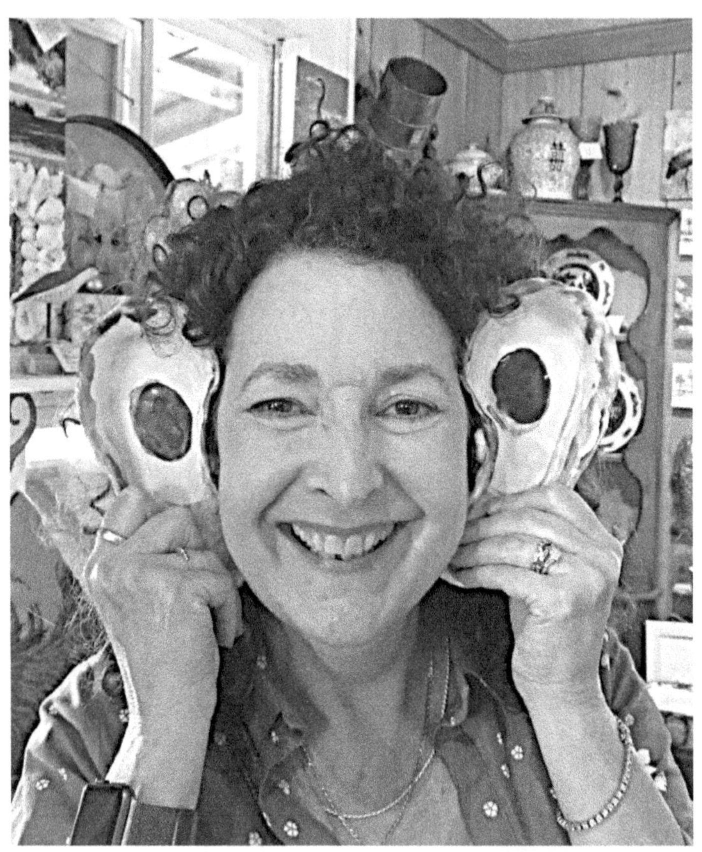

Me on vacation-always finding “EARS”.

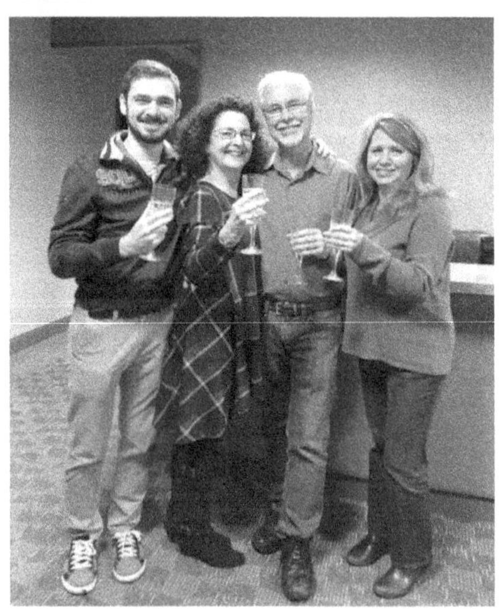

This picture was taken when we celebrated moving into our current location in 2016. Pictured left from right is our son Zach, who worked with us at the time, myself, my husband, John and our fabulous front office manager, Lisa.

ABOUT THE AUTHOR

DR. JEWELL IS AN EXPERT IN AUDIOLOGY with a Master's degree from LSU Medical Center in New Orleans and a doctoral degree from AT Still University in Arizona. She is a published author in the American Journal of Otolaryngology (2009), co-authoring a paper on the use of micronutrients in the treatment of tinnitus. She has been a member of both audiology professional organizations (AAA and ADA), served on both the AAA Ethical Practices Committee and on the Ethical Practices Committee for the Tennessee Academy of Speech-Language Pathology and Audiology organization. She has been awarded the AAA scholar award for several consecutive years for her dedication to continuing education. She also served as the Private Practice Representative and President for the Tennessee Academy of Audiology and contributed to re-writing Tennessee state guidelines for both audiologists and hearing instrument specialists. Dr. Jewell's clinical experience is varied, including ENT practices, a school system, hearing aid manufacturers, and in clinical private practice. She is the owner of Audiology and Hearing Health (est. 1992) where her husband, John, serves as practice manager and hearing instrument specialist.

She has presented at professional conferences throughout her career and is always happy to present at local organizations to promote healthy hearing. She is also a Certified Dementia Practitioner through the National Council of Certified Dementia Practitioners (NCCDP). This additional certification demonstrates achievement and specialized training in the areas of Alzheimer's and dementia care.

On a personal note, Dr. Jewell and her husband have one son, (Zach, married to his high school sweetheart, Jordan), three dogs, and one cat. They love to vacation together - favorites places are South Carolina beaches, Louisiana, and Lake Tahoe. She is a proud member of a competition a Capella chorus (Metro Nashville Chorus) and has performed with them in regional and national competitions and even on the stage of the famous Ryman Auditorium in Nashville, TN.

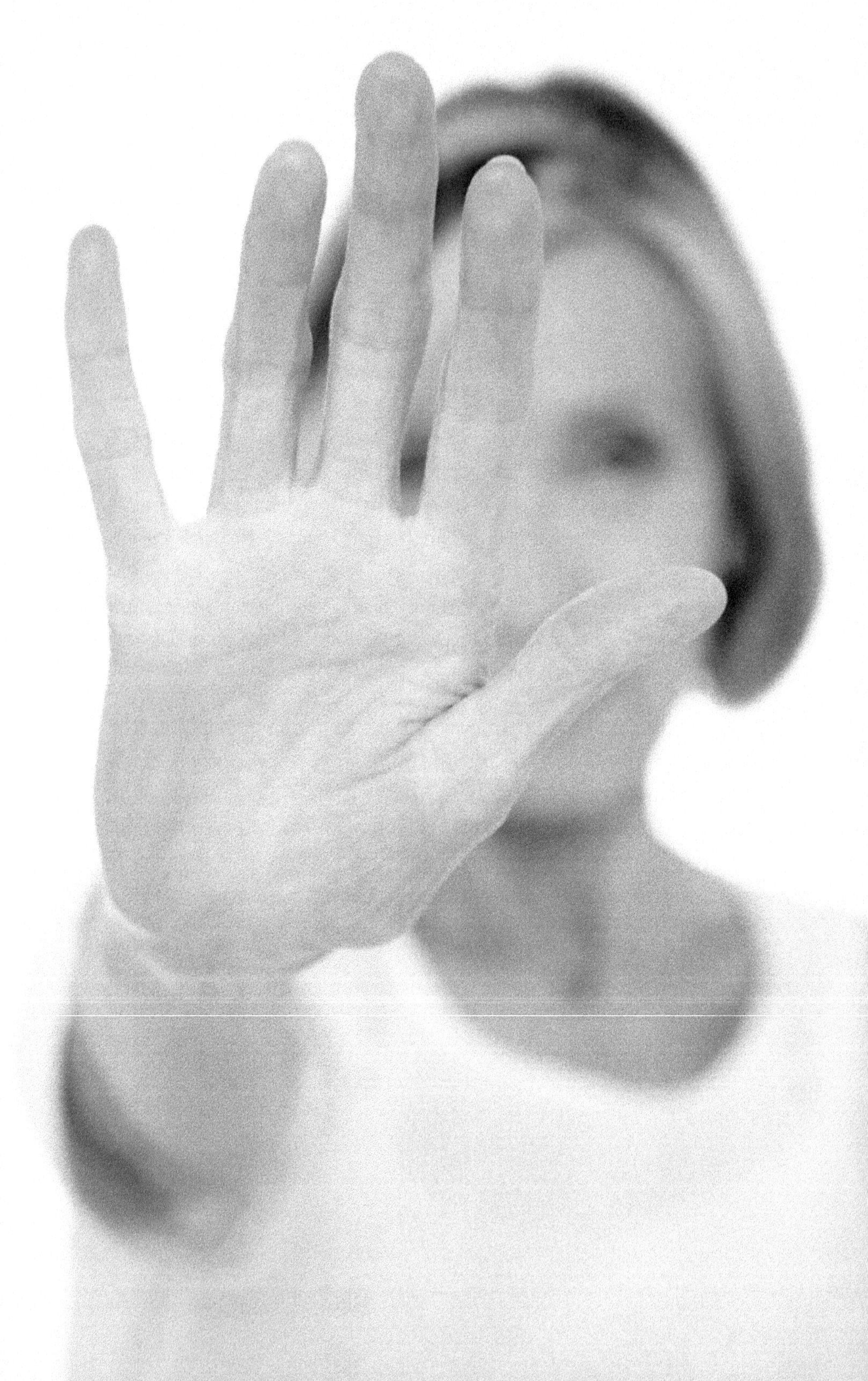

INTRODUCTION

The Top 5 Reasons People Avoid Seeing a Hearing Care Specialist

My name is Dr. Jewell Baggett-Strehlau, and I'm a private practice audiologist. When people hear what I do for a living, they almost always say, "huh?". It's just too hard to resist! It's okay; it does help to break the ice.

The fact is, the less you know about audiology and treating hearing loss, the more reason you have to be afraid of it. Once upon a time, hearing aids meant one thing: big, heavy, ugly "beige bananas" to be worn on your ear to make sounds louder. They were hard to put on, hard to adjust, and frankly, they were pretty terrible at doing anything other than making all sounds louder…this includes speech, background noise, loud ventilation machines, dogs barking, plates clanging, etc.!

For the majority of patients, wearing an old-fashioned hearing aid meant avoiding certain social situations, restaurants, family gatherings playing with grandchildren, etc. Many people still cling to the unfounded notion that all hearing aids are created equal and perform the same way they did back in 1982! I was just getting started back then.... I remember those things.

The fact of the matter is that audiology and the clinical science of treating hearing loss is more than just hearing aids. How much more?

Audiology and the medical treatment of hearing loss is devoted to restoring an individual's clarity, restoring personal independence, improving cognitive function and mental health, and addressing the cognitive aspects of hearing loss that can increase the risk of developing dementia.

Maintaining proper hearing and cognitive health has a significant impact on an individual's life—including all of his or her family, friends, and community members. Properly stimulating cognitive function and maintaining connections from the ear to the brain goes a long way in keeping a patient mentally competent, helping the patient remain autonomous, and helping keep at bay the mind robbing diseases associated with cognitive decline (i.e., Alzheimer's). Treating hearing loss is a wonderful investment with lifelong returns, and yet people still fear walking into a hearing health care provider's office for one simple reason—fear of the unknown!

Hey—it's okay to be worried about the unknown. We all have our reasons for avoiding a visit to the doctor.

For many, visiting a doctor of audiology is accompanied by many fears and anxieties. And for each patient, the experience is personal. There are reasons that patients typically wait seven years before being seen by a doctor of audiology and beginning treatment of their hearing loss. This list, Top 5 Reasons People Avoid Seeing a Hearing Care Specialist, has the most common conversations I have had with patients over the years about what took them so long to come into my office.

It is important to remember that the consequences of un-treated hearing loss can negatively impact every part of your life, even making you dependent on others and at a significantly increased risk of developing dementia.

REASON #1 – The Patient Already Knows the Diagnosis Before He or She Ever Steps Foot in the Door.

Individuals with hearing loss tend to wait nearly seven years before raising their hand and admitting they have a problem. Or perhaps it takes a family member nearly seven years to push his or her loved one through our office door! Either way, seven seems to be the "unlucky" number—I say "unlucky" because chances are very high that by the seventh year of experiencing the symptoms of hearing loss, significant damage has been done to the auditory system, which can lower treatment outcomes. I try to explain to all of my patients that hearing loss is a progressive degenerative disorder with neurologic involvement which undoubtedly requires early intervention. In lay terms, that simply means that your hearing will continue to degrade as you age, and the key to maintaining clarity and a higher level of hearing function (i.e., hearing in noisy environments) is to "catch it early and treat it early."

I have empathy for the new patient who comes to my office to get his or her first hearing evaluation since grade school because I know, as does the patient, what the results will likely be. It is very brave for a patient to knowingly enter a medical office with the understanding that he or she is likely to receive the diagnosis of progressive degenerative age-related hearing loss. Especially a disorder that is neither reversible, nor is there a cure. However, there are restorative treatments available that can help the patient stay connected at home, at work, in their community and that can help stimulate the brain, improving cognitive function, and even reduce the risk of developing dementia (more on the connections of hearing loss and dementia later in the book!).

REASON #2 – The Patient is Not Sure of His or Her Insurance Coverage for the Procedures and Treatments Involved with Hearing Loss.

Regardless of when you read this book and which administration is running our country, insurance is a complex world to attempt to muddle through, and when it comes to hearing health care coverage, it can be even more murky. BUT...nearly every insurance company I have come across allows for coverage of one diagnostic hearing evaluation per year by an audiologist (and more testing can be covered if medically necessary, i.e., if the patient notices a significant sudden change in hearing). A hearing evaluation is often considered "preventative" and, in many cases, does not require a referral from your physician.

While it is nearly impossible to speak for every patient and every insurance plan, this is intended to help ease the stress of navigating the process of hearing health care coverage. In fact, I believe any reputable hearing health care practice will have a deep understanding of the insurance regulations in its area and will be able to readily answer any questions you may have about your insurance coverage—or at least be willing to help you find the answer.

In my many years of experience in the hearing health care field, I have watched firsthand as patient benefits for treatment of hearing loss have evolved—fortunately, in a direction that benefits the patient. Yes, medical treatment of your hearing loss may have an out-of-pocket cost associated with it, but I have seen insurance cover anywhere from 10% to 100% of the costs. And even if you were in the position of having 0% insurance coverage, treating hearing loss can be affordable—and you will learn throughout this book that treating hearing loss is truly priceless and can hardly be assigned a monetary value.

REASON #3 – Patients are Afraid of Being Sold Something.

It's like magic—once you turn the respectful age of sixty, you notice that the content of your mailbox seems to change. Nearly every week, perhaps a few times a week, you are fortunate (I'm being sarcastic, here) to have a full mailbox (both your physical and electronic mailbox) with literature about "essential vitamins for seniors," "how to choose the right assisted living residence," "how to invest your retirement money," "join AARP," and "which digital technology widget is best for your hearing loss." YIKES!

Somewhere along the line, hearing health care started down the dangerous road of becoming a retail transaction. I've even seen some so-called hearing widgets sold at big-box retailers and chain pharmacies… Like I ask my patients: "If a colonoscopy was available at one of the big-box chains, would you take your loved one there to have it done? NO…so why would you treat your hearing loss there?". It is certainly easy, "free hearing test" and all, but the nature of a big-box store does not allow for the gold standard of care that everyone deserves. There is so much misinformation out there, I don't blame the patient for sometimes entering the office thinking he/she is going to be "sold" something.

My best advice is to steer clear of anybody trying to sell you something (be wary anytime the hearing test is "free"). If we go back to Reason #1 above, the patient is likely already nervous because he or she knows the medical diagnosis before ever even stepping foot in the office. Combine that with the fear of "being sold something" and that makes for a pretty nervous patient with his or her guard up.

Unfortunately, much of modern medicine is turning into a commercial advertisement seen on TV that marginalizes the process of treating a medical disorder, and hearing health care is not immune to this. In my office, and in other Audigy member-clinics across the country, our belief is in the medical evaluation and treatment of hearing loss.

I believe strongly that the proper medical treatment of hearing loss is best left to the clinicians specially trained to understand, diagnose, and treat your hearing loss.

REASON #4 – The Cost.

Actual Cost

We all know somebody, perhaps a family member or a friend, who has spent a significant amount of money on a hearing aid gizmo only to use it as a paperweight or to leave it in his or her sock drawer. And the reason is because the glorified over-priced amplifier that he or she purchased was never truly designed to improve hearing or clarity—it was designed to just make sounds louder. This truly angers me, and while I do believe that the patient plays a significant role in his or her healthcare decisions and follow-up care, the health care provider also must have a significant responsibility to the patient—even after the patient has left the office.

I have heard too many horror stories about patients spending upwards of $10,000.00 on a pair of hearing aid gizmos. More often than not, this very high retail transaction very likely took place in one of the chain hearing aid sales shops with "free hearing tests" that advertise in the newspaper or on TV.

I will refrain from mentioning the names of these well-known offenders that use misleading advertisements and high pressure sales techniques. Sadly, all the patients got in return for their money were hearing aids capable of making things louder.

When a practice and the providers are committed to the medical treatment of hearing loss, you can trust that you are in good hands.

I believe that a hearing specialist must meet the strict standards required of Audigy member-clinics and follow the medical model of treating hearing loss.

I have always believed that the patient needs options to help him or her invest in proper hearing health care. A reputable audiology practice understands that for some people, the upfront investment in hearing healthcare can be prohibitive. Patients must be provided with options. All Audigy member-clinics will offer reputable creditors/banks to help establish a payment plan (some with 0% interest for up to 18 months, or even a longer-term payment plan with fixed interest rates). Recently we discovered an affordable subscription plan that will be offered at my clinic which provides individuals with the opportunity to pay a one-time down payment and a small monthly fee thereafter with the advantage of full warranty (loss, damage, and repair coverage for life), complete access to supplies, batteries and service appointments for life, and no-cost automatic upgrades in NeuroTechnology™ for life.

Hidden Cost

What about the cost of not treating hearing loss? While research has yet to make the definitive finding that hearing loss can cause dementia (causality is often difficult in clinical science), the evidence that the relationship exists is overwhelming. Even more important is the mounting evidence that treating hearing loss may significantly reduce the risk of developing dementia.

Every day, 10,000 people turn sixty-five years young. This trend is expected to continue for at least the next fifteen years. And it is almost a guarantee that over the next fifteen years, science will continue to reduce the mortality rate and increase the average life expectancy. As a result, our health care system will be pushed to its capacity to deal with diseases such as cancer, diabetes, cardiovascular disease, etc.

Perhaps the most prevalent, most costly, and most disabling of all diseases we will see sharply rise over the ensuing decades is dementia—the mind-robbing mental disease that interrupts and interferes with every aspect of life. Dementia is not a normal part of aging.

Every three to four seconds, another patient is diagnosed with dementia. Rates of dementia are estimated to triple in the next thirty years. Unlike the other diseases listed above, a physical body with dementia is estimated to outlive the individual's mental capabilities by ten or more years! It is estimated that the average cost, per family, to manage the medical treatment and care of a loved one with dementia can exceed $57,000.00 per year.

There is no cure for this catastrophic disease, but there are treatments available, including several ways to decrease your risk of developing dementia. **In fact, a study published in The Lancet journal indicated that the treatment of hearing loss is the single most modifiable factor in the prevention of dementia.**

I encourage you to read a report detailing "9 Key Lifestyle Tips to Reduce the Risk of Developing Dementia." This report can be found at ***www.ExcellenceInAudiology.org.***

REASON #5 – Nobody LIKES Hearing Aids.

Let's be honest. Nobody likes hearing aids. In fact, when you make a reference to old-fashioned volume-enhancing hearing aids, I think you could go so far as to say, "some hearing aids are horrible!" There you have it—I said it! I've been working with hearing-impaired patients for close to forty years and although my patients love improved hearing, they might not love their hearing aids. I don't see a reason to tip-toe around this subject or ignore the fact that patients generally do not like using hearing aids. Nobody wants a medical disorder that requires physically tethering a device to his or her body to treat the medical condition. They don't like their glasses either, but they do like to be able to see! (Although I do know some people who wear non-prescriptive glasses because they feel that they look "cool"). I remember growing up in a time where people who wore glasses were sometimes referred to as "four-eyes" or other derogatory terms—fortunately glasses are now commonplace for people of all ages. I started wearing glasses at the age of twelve and trust me, I did NOT look cool. But I did like being able to see the leaves on trees. Who knew??

For some people, hearing aids carry the stigma of meaning "I'm old and ready to die." And nearly every day I see a patient try to tell him or herself not to invest in hearing health care treatment because "eh, I won't be around much longer anyway." My response is always the same-to ask them about the quality of life they want to experience and if they want to remain connected to their loved ones and the world around them. No matter if they live for a few more years, or even thirty more years (which is not unreasonable to expect from my fifty-eight-year young patients), isn't it worth wanting to hear and understand everything and everyone else in your life? I also point out to patients that they will appear to look much older if they continue to say "what?" or "huh?" all the time or, perhaps even worse, start to isolate themselves from life and the conversations around them.

I get it, and I respect that patients don't want to use a hearing aid, whatever the reason may be. I use Neuro-Technology hearing aids myself for treatment of my tinnitus. Sometimes I don't want to wear them, but it helps my tinnitus, so I do. Any reputable hearing health care provider will realize this also and understand the difference between traditional hearing aids and advanced NeuroTechnology™. Features in NeuroTechnology™ are specifically designed to treat the medical condition of hearing loss, improve cognitive function, and improve overall quality of life. As an added benefit, NeuroTechnology™ is incredibly discrete and comes in several invisible styles (more on invisible hearing-loss treatment options later in the book).

PART 1

FINDING A HEARING HEALTH CARE SPECIALIST

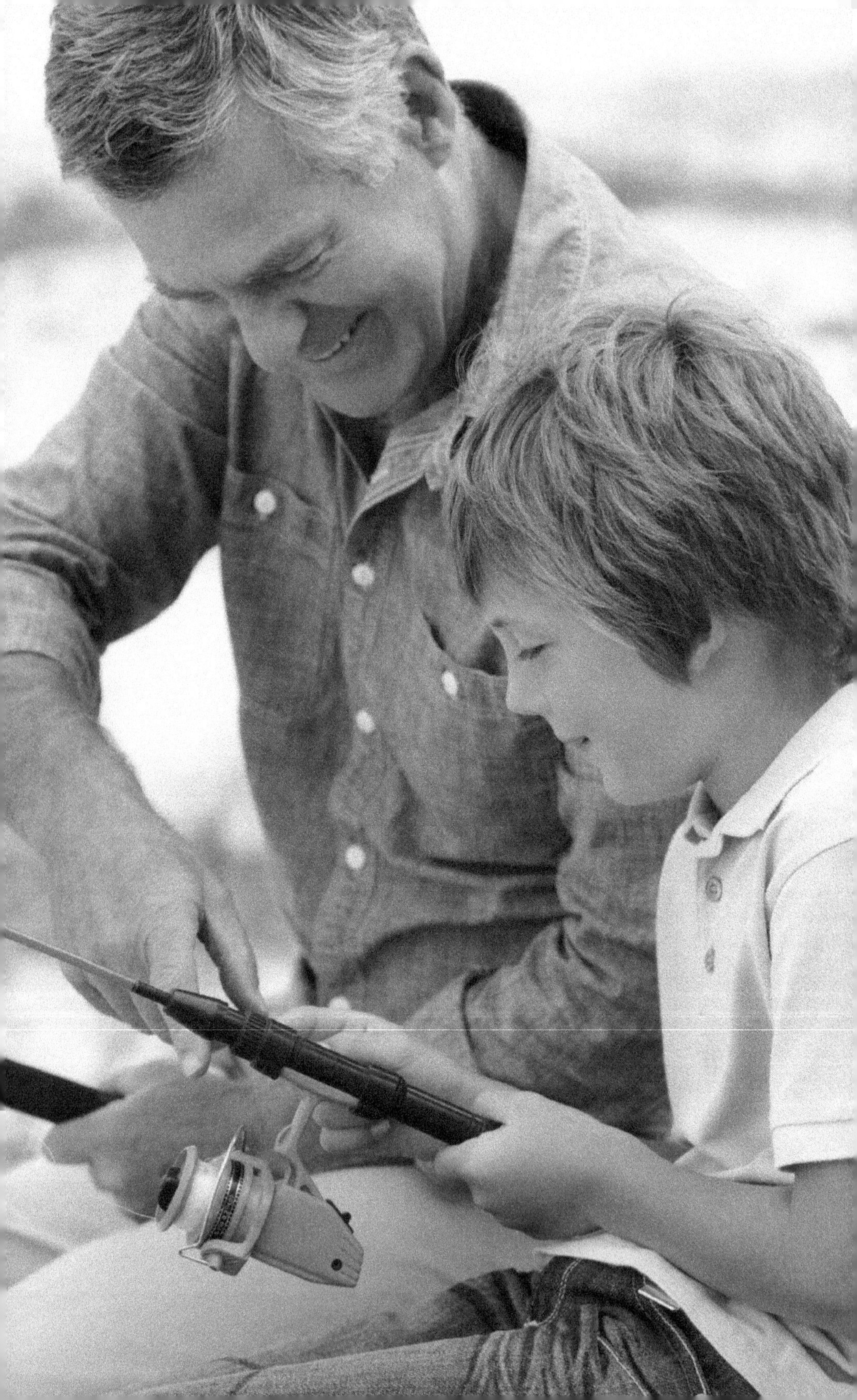

QUESTION #1

Why is hearing so important?

I believe most people can relate to my story: I saw from afar my dear stepfather degrade as he crossed over from his seventies to his eighties. As he got older, his hearing got worse—and as the hearing got worse, his cognitive abilities declined. His hearing aid use was inconsistent, and he lost more than one pair. As a result, our ability to communicate with him was significantly affected. Although I had seen similar patients in my practice, this was my first personal experience with hearing loss being correlated to cognitive decline (AKA dementia). It's a lot harder when it happens to someone you love.

Communication is truly the basic building block of every relationship we have at work, at home with our loved ones, with our children, etc. Communication is a vital part of establishing and maintaining relationships. Watching my stepfather decline helped push me to be a better student, a better teacher, and a better clinician. As I started seeing more and more patients with dementia and saw how the use of good hearing systems helped them, I wanted to learn more about how hearing loss and cognitive decline were related. That knowledge has allowed me to advance my patients' care to the highest level and to understand new standards for testing and treatment protocol used in clinics across the country.

QUESTION #2

What are some of the early signs of hearing loss, and when should I see a specialist?

Hearing loss is typically a slow, gradual onset disorder that silently (pardon the pun) affects the individual. The most common symptoms experienced by most (perhaps not all) patients are difficulty hearing in background noise, tinnitus, and thinking most people mumble or speak too softly. They say, "if others wouldn't mumble, I'd hear them just fine!" Most people who experience the initial symptoms of hearing loss do not even realize it is happening. It is far easier to blame the acoustics of the room, the volume of the background noise, or the person speaking (i.e., "they mumble") than it is to accept that it's your hearing that has changed. It is also difficult for many patients to rationalize the need for medical treatment of hearing loss because in some (ideal listening) situations (i.e., sitting at a table one-on-one in a perfectly quiet environment) may not be much of a challenge. But the truth is…

A Mild Hearing Loss is a Major Problem!

The first symptom of hearing loss for most patients is difficulty hearing in complex listening environments. If you have this issue, take the time to reflect truly and deeply on your communication breakdown. I believe you will begin to recognize some of the initial symptoms of hearing loss. Are you having any difficulty when there are a few people at the kitchen table? Or when the kids come over? Or when communicating with your grandchildren? Or when you are at a social gathering (i.e., sharing a meal with friends and you can't seem to follow the conversation, yet all the other people seem to be enjoying themselves and following the conversation)? It is in these types of scenarios when hearing loss can really start to affect your ability to understand and you realize that you are no longer an active part of the conversation. The result is a slow retraction from contributing to the conversation because you may feel embarrassed, and thus you continue to further isolate yourself and find yourself not truly engaging in conversations and relationships. And this is how even a mild hearing loss can really begin to impact your quality of life and relationships with others.

In addition to the importance of maintaining an active, engaged life with family and friends, early treatment of mild hearing loss is important for maintaining proper brain health. Simply put: Hearing Care is Health Care™. Your hearing drives your conception of everything and everybody around you; thus, hearing is essentially driving cognition at all times. It's driving memory. It's driving your image of the environment around you. You don't turn hearing on or off; you can't close your ears like you can close your eyes. There really isn't a sense or portion of your brain that isn't connected to your auditory system.

And I believe this speaks to how important hearing is to live and to thrive. We are bombarded with sound at all times and the brain is constantly, in real-time, making decisions as to whether or not certain sounds are important, trying to figure out how to categorize the sound and if it is important to store away and remember it for reference at a later date. A mild hearing loss can take away significant portions of the auditory world around you—and can even be related to why patients with untreated hearing loss are at a significantly higher risk of experiencing a devastating fall.

The lack of cognitive stimulation that accompanies even a mild hearing loss is also associated with cognitive decline and dementia. Reports from Johns Hopkins Medical Center (and others) indicate that a mild hearing loss can increase the risk of developing dementia by 200% (up to a 500% increase for those with a severe hearing loss).

Like every major medical condition, the key to successful management of the disorder is early intervention.

"Catch it early and treat it early!"

QUESTION #3

Why, and how, should I choose a specialist for my hearing loss treatment?

I get this question so often that I developed a Top 10 List (although it's not nearly as fun as David Letterman's Top 10 Lists). This list can help a patient understand "why" they need to choose a specialist and "how" to choose the right specialist to trust with the treatment of their hearing loss.

The Top 10 Things You Must Know before Choosing Your Hearing Health Care Provider

❶ Is He or She a Specialist?

Hearing health care consists of both audiologists and hearing instrument specialists; both working towards the same goal—to help more people struggling with hearing loss. Audiologists are clinically trained hearing health care specialists with doctoral degrees that require several extra years of training in order to provide the most thorough diagnostic evaluation and complete the most comprehensive treatment plans aimed at restoring hearing clarity. They are typically located in medical-type offices and are able to bill health insurance for diagnostic exams. Hearing instrument specialist are trained to give basic hearing tests and dispense hearing aids. They are typically located in retail-type stores that offer "free" hearing tests (for the purpose of hearing aid selection and sales-and not billed to insurance).

Audiologists are hearing health care providers that perform auditory diagnostics, counseling, and rehabilitation, which is likely to include the use of Neuro-Technology™ that provides proper stimulation to the auditory system. This is a fancy way to describe how we normalize the way our brains process the incoming sounds in order to achieve maximum clarity, especially in background noise.

Another sign of a great specialist is he or she can tell you about a before and after scenario of a similar case that he or she has previously helped. We know all ears are different, but with the 100,000+ ears our Audigy member-clinics have restored clarity to, we can tell you about a similar case to your specific hearing situation.

❷ Does the Hearing Health Care Provider Have a Medical Office (or a Sales Office)?

In the hearing aid world, it is not hard to open up shop on a shoestring budget and call yourself a specialist. When you are searching for a provider, make sure you understand the clinician's credentials and medical affiliations. Often times, smaller offices with limited staff with non-audiology providers are somewhat limited in their service offerings and stability.

If you find a hearing care provider with the best credentials and an office that is inviting and in a medical setting, you have found a specialist who understands the importance of hearing health care and will be around for years to come to help you and your family best understand and address your hearing needs.

Audigy member-clinics are located across the country with hearing health care clinicians of the highest caliber who insist on the best practice (often setting the standards for best practices) for their patients and loved ones.

❸ Does the Specialist Think Brain First?

Everybody thinks "we hear with our ears," and while that is partially correct, the process of hearing actually happens at the level of the brain. Today's hearing loss treatments are far more than a simple "amplifying" device behind your ear. The neuroscience behind modern treatments is focused on the brain, cognition, and the comorbidities of untreated hearing loss (comorbidity is defined as a disorder that co-occurs/is correlated to hearing loss). If your clinician thinks hearing first and not brain first in his or her treatment plan, you are missing out on many long-term lifestyle benefits. NeuroTechnology™ is aimed at restoring lost clarity, providing noise-canceling filters for noisy background situations, and soft-speech enhancers that emphasize the speech of those soft-speakers in your life.

When searching for your hearing health care provider, make sure you find a specialist that understands the significant negative impacts of untreated hearing loss on your brain. To find a local clinician who has been recognized for their commitment to thinking brain first in treatment plans, prescriptions, and protocols, you can visit the website ***www.agxhearing.com*.**

❹ Do They Include a Technology Demonstration After Diagnostics are Completed?

Most audiologists offer no-obligation demonstrations of technology for new patients so that you and your family can get expert advice about treatment needs, options, and timing before making this important investment.

During your first evaluation and consultation, be sure your questions are being answered, your concerns are being addressed, and you are being educated about all your treatment options. The clinician should include a comprehensive written report during, or after, the evaluation at no charge.

❺ Does the Provider's Office Offer an Evaluation Period with a Comprehensive Treatment Plan?

No matter which hearing health care provider you choose, ultimately you are not making a small investment—in both time and finances. That being said, it is important to know that your clinician is going to stand behind his or her medical treatment plan. Every Audigy member-clinic offers multiple assurances that you have chosen the right provider and the right treatment plan.

Be sure your provider offers a plan that covers cleaning services, office visits, repairs, and prescriptive programming. A typical plan is one year, but because we follow a gold standard of hearing care, we provide three years of coverage in our treatment plan, including loss and damage coverage for our patients.

Rest assured—your hearing health care is my priority. Thus, I stand by everything I've recommended in this publication.

❻ Is He or She Using the Latest Technology and Treatment Options Available?

Audiology today differs a great deal from years past. Computer-designed NeuroTechnology™ devices and wireless technologies dramatically increase the precision with which we restore clarity and boost hearing ability. Scientific verification of device settings, while in your ear (referred to as Real Ear Measurements) maximize the precision of NeuroTechnology™ benefits. As an added incentive, today's NeuroTechnology™ are discrete and virtually undetectable to the user and others. In fact, a new category of NeuroTechnology™, known for being invisible, can offer the most discrete, cosmetically pleasing option placed deep in your ear canal to make the entire treatment a well-kept secret!

❼ Does Your Investment Include Treatment Supplies?

Each hearing care office has its own fee schedules, and specialists often charge differently for procedures. All specialists should offer you a contract which clearly spells out the investment for you or your loved one's treatment before it begins.

❽ Does the Specialist Charge for Follow-Up and Emergency Appointments?

Each time a patient embarks on the journey of improved hearing, there is an adaptation period for the user's ears and brain to adjust. This period can take thirty to forty-five days and is individual to each patient. In addition to the complex cognitive changes that happen when restoring hearing clarity, patients will notice significant improvement in some hearing situations and perhaps not as much in some other situations. This is common in the initial process of hearing loss treatments. I believe every patient is entitled to ongoing customizations for their NeuroTechnology™ prescription throughout their treatment plan.

Keep in mind, if your NeuroTechnology™ is broken or damaged due to non-compliance with care, protection, and maintenance, this may result in repair charges. As a simple rule, if you do your best to avoid breaking your NeuroTechnology™ and follow the simple guidelines that your audiology specialist shares with you, then you should have no additional costs for customizations, even if it's an "emergency."

⑨ Does the Clinician Make You Feel Special and Comfortable?

When you meet with your hearing health care provider, the person you are trusting with your hearing health care, you need to be in a comfortable and welcoming environment. Each employee in my clinic understands the importance of hearing and the distress that can be involved with making the decision to treat one's hearing loss. In fact, several members of my staff wear hearing devices themselves (myself included)! The entire experience from beginning to end, including a welcoming staff, should be designed to help alleviate a person's feelings of anxiety or grief.

We believe every patient is special and must be made to feel that way every time he or she comes to one of our offices in need of hearing health care.

⑩ Does the Specialist Have a Great Reputation?

With the internet today, it is extremely easy to pull up ratings and reviews from patients. Simply go to Google and search for audiology reviews and ratings within your town. At the time of this report, my practice has multiple five-star reviews on Google, Facebook, and other online sources. And don't be shy about asking for references—go directly to the source! You have the right to call any audiology office and ask for a list of references, including other patients and local physicians that have volunteered to help advise patients as they first enter the (sometimes overwhelming) world of hearing loss and to help patients understand rehabilitation experiences from the first person perspective.

QUESTION #4

How early in life should I have my hearing evaluated?

The Simple Answer

If you are over fifty, you should have your hearing evaluated.

Detailed Answer

I have tried to stress the importance of early diagnosis and treatment of hearing loss throughout this book and to each of my patients.

The American Speech Language Hearing Association, the American Academy of Audiology and the American Medical Association have all considered the recommendation of including "hearing evaluation/screening" between the ages of fifty to sixty years young. I have used the catch phrase "Ears and Rears" as my way of getting people to remember to have their hearing checked when they turn fifty (and of course, have a colon cancer screening too!).

Similar to going to your primary care physician every year, obtaining a baseline hearing test can help to better serve you and your clinician as a guide to the medical recommendation at current or future appointments. Obtaining a baseline evaluation and discovering that you have normal hearing never hurt anyone!

Regardless of age, if you are noticing any of the symptoms of hearing loss (e.g., difficulty hearing in noisy situations, difficulty hearing the TV compared to others), if your family is suggesting you get a hearing test, or if you have ringing in your ears (defined as tinnitus), then it is time to take the first step and have your hearing evaluated and discuss treatment options.

Unfortunately, waiting too long can significantly impact the expectations and outcome of treatment, and sadly every hearing health care clinician I know has a patient they have had to tell he or she waited too long, and the benefits of treatment will be minimal.

PART 2
FIXING THE RIGHT THINGS AT THE RIGHT TIME

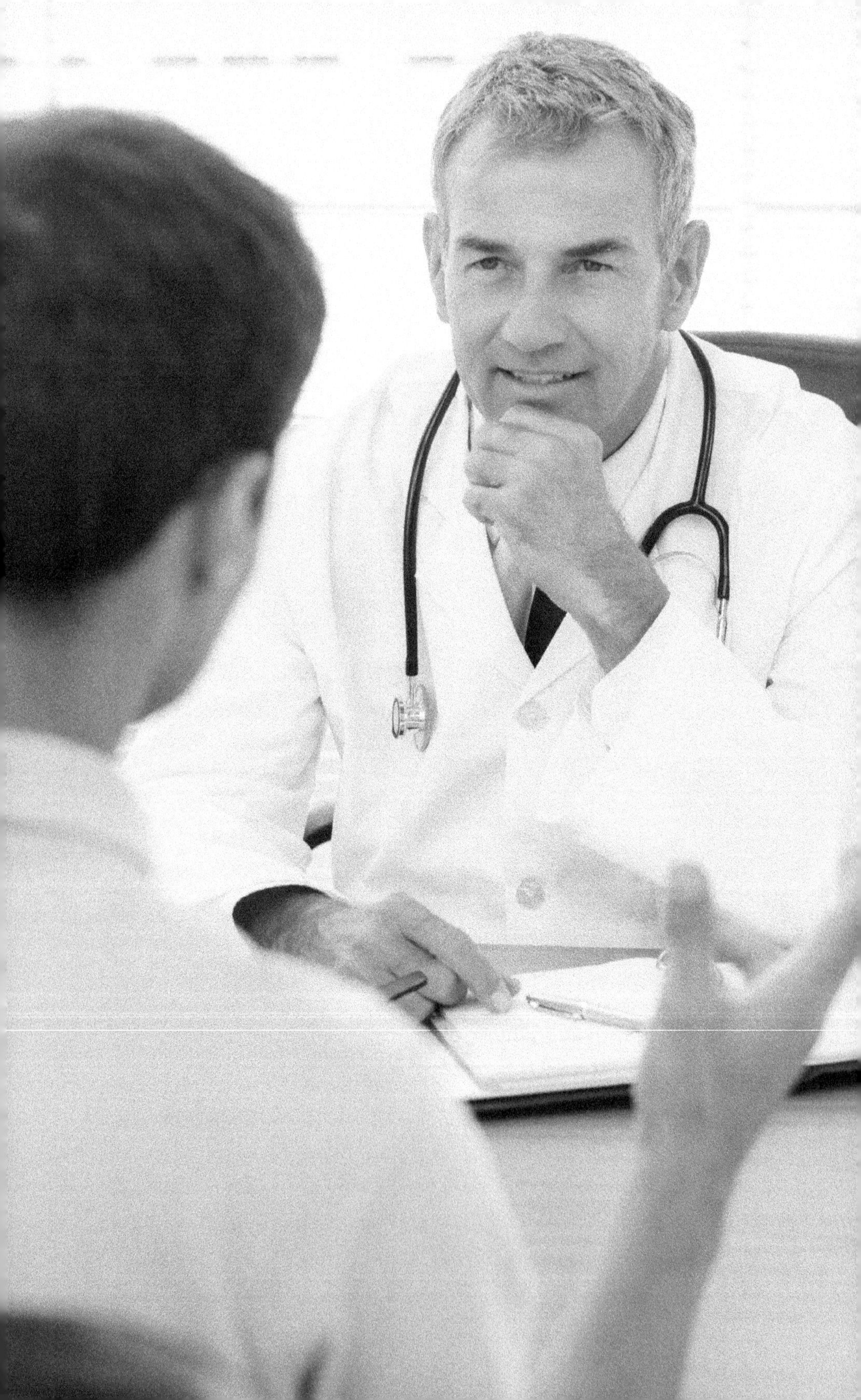

QUESTION #5

What will happen at the initial evaluation and consultation?

Every process has a beginning, middle, and end.

The Beginning

First things first…your specialist will ask you "So, tell me, what is going on with your ears?" (or some variation of that "why" question). This helps to set the stage for understanding your specific hearing related issues, concerns, and experiences. This conversation is the baseline to helping your audiologist understand why you "raised your hand and are seeking help." While my job title may be "audiologist," this initial line of questioning is designed to help me better understand my patient at a deeper, more emotional level. I want to know my patient's experience with hearing loss and how it impacts his/her life. How does your hearing loss impact your relationship with your children or grandchildren? How does hearing loss impact your relationship with your spouse? Does hearing loss get in the way of your performance at work? Some of my patients wait for years to be able to go fishing with their grandchild, and now their hearing loss is robbing them of the richness of that experience and getting in the way of developing a deeper relationship. As an audiologist, it is my job to treat your hearing loss and you as a person.

The Middle

Treating hearing loss is a process steeped in science, engineering, technology, and clinical medicine. There is also an "art" to treating hearing loss, and this skill is developed with years of experience. In order to develop the right treatment plan for each patient, first there must be the proper diagnostic procedures that tests every aspect of hearing.

HOW DOES THE EAR WORK?

So, because I am the EarNerd, I always want to be sure patients understand how their ears work. It is our ears' job to take in acoustic sound waves (all the sounds around us travel in invisible sound waves) and turn them into electricity which is how our brain and nervous system communicate. Sound goes into and makes the eardrum vibrate. This is where the first energy change happens.

When the eardrum vibrates, the acoustic energy changes to mechanical energy. The tiny bones attached to the eardrum also vibrate and send the energy into the inner ear (the cochlea). The inner ear is a tiny, fluid-filled space inside the temporal bone (remember, the hardest bone in the human body?). The inner ear is so small, the whole thing could fit on my pinky fingernail bed. As fluid is moving, the energy is now hydraulic, which causes the tiny "hair cells" to move inside the inner ear in the same fashion that seaweed moves in ocean tides. That movement makes the final change to electricity which then travels up the hearing nerve, (8th cranial nerve) and then to the auditory centers of the brain. How cool is that? Sound that goes into the right ear ends up in the left side of the brain, while sound going into the left ear goes to the right side of the brain, then the energy crosses over from each side to the other side. That is how our brain tells where sound is coming from, and also helps us process speech in the presence of noise.

What am amazing process, and it all happens in milliseconds!! SO COOL!

Everything that I do in the exam is analyzing how the sound is moving through all of the above processes so that I can figure out if there is a loss of energy somewhere that is resulting in your loss of hearing. If the problem is earwax, that can be removed. If the problem is in the middle ear, there may be medical or surgical treatments that are appropriate for you. If the problem is that the inner ear hair cells are damaged, then you just may need some extra sound stimulation that will help your brain get the sound that it is missing. This is why it is so important that you see a clinical audiologist so that your hearing loss is properly evaluated. In my many years of practice, I have unfortunately seen many patients that were "sold" hearing aids when their hearing loss could have been medically or surgically corrected.

So, now that I have geeked out, onto the exam. First, your audiologist will look into the ear canal to make sure the ears are not blocked with cerumen (ear wax). This is most often followed by a procedure called tympanometry that can rule out medical conditions causing hearing loss involving the eardrum and/or the space behind it, including those tiny, middle ear bones (the "Hammer, Anvil, and Stirrup").

The Beeps!

From there, it is important to establish the degree of hearing loss (ranked from mild to profound). Using the "raise your hand when you hear the beep" may conjure memories of having your hearing screened by the school nurse, but it still serves a purpose: establishing the degree of hearing loss. If the person stops testing you after the beeps and makes a recommendation for treating your hearing loss…I advise you to run as fast as you can! The information gathered from this test, although important, is only a piece of the puzzle.

The Words!

The most important testing we will perform is designed to assess your cognitive hearing, e.g., how well you understand words in quiet and with background noise (after all, nobody comes to the office complaining that they can't hear beeps!). This part will truly help your clinician understand how well you process words and conversation.

Testing a patient's ability to hear words is often referred to as "Word Discrimination Scores/Ability." First the patient is asked to repeat a list of words at a near-normal conversational volume. Individuals with normal hearing will always correctly repeat between 96-100% of the words on this test. Individuals with hearing loss will not score nearly as well. For example, many people with a mild to moderate hearing age-related hearing loss will typically score between 50-60%—thus the patient is expected to miss 40-50% of what is said to him or her on a daily basis (especially when visual and contextual cues are removed and only hearing is utilized).

The next test is a repeat, almost exactly as just described, but performed a second time at a volume and clarity setting ideal for the specific patient's hearing loss. The result of this second round of word testing is referred to as the patient's "Hearing Potential Score." Most often the patient who formerly scored between 50-60% will now score 90% and greater; thus, treatment with NeuroTechnology™ is expected to improve the patient's hearing clarity to 90% and greater on a daily basis (especially in a quiet conversational setting). The patient is fully aware that he or she performed significantly better with enhanced clarity.

I mentioned earlier that the consequences of waiting too long to treat hearing loss can be dire. In some cases when the second round of word testing is completed, the patient's "Hearing Potential Score" will sometimes only be as high as 50-60%. In these cases, the outcomes and expectations for treatment are very dim (especially when compared with the patient who scored over 90%).

The Words In Background Noise!

The #1 complaint of every patient with hearing loss, and most often the first symptom of hearing loss, is difficulty understanding speech and conversation in background noise. Thus, it is critical that the clinician understands each patient's ability to decipher speech in background noise (again, without visual or contextual cues). This test, called the Quick Speech in Noise Test (QuickSIN™), is a means to quantify a patient's difficulty understanding and following speech in background noise.

Briefly, the sentence intended to be heard and repeated by the listener is presented at a clear and audible volume to the patient. With each new sentence introduced, the level of background noise (often referred to as "cocktail party noise") is increased in increments of five decibels. The final iteration of the test is when the speech and background "babble" are presented at the same volume— significantly taxing the auditory system and its noise-reduction filters.

Individuals with normal hearing are typically capable of hearing every word at each level, and some of the words at the final, most competitive level. In contrast, individuals with even a mild hearing loss can struggle significantly on this test when the noise is ten decibels less than the intended speech. The test is scored on a Hearing Handicap Scale and can range from normal, to mild, to moderate, to severe hearing handicap. A majority of patients with a mild age-related hearing loss will often score in the mild to moderate hearing handicap range, confirming his or her reported difficulty following conversation in complex listening situations.

The End

Once all the testing is complete, it is the clinician's responsibility to review all test results with the patient and with his or her loved ones. These results are personal and can help a patient better understand the difficulty he or she is dealing with on a daily basis. Understanding the results can also be just as important for family and loved ones.

Although an individual with normal hearing can only imagine what it feels like to suffer from permanent hearing loss, gaining an understanding of the degree of hearing loss, hearing potential ability, and hearing handicap scores can help the loved ones gain perspective on what the patient is going through and how much of a strain hearing loss can be.

These test results will determine the medical treatment plan and help initiate the journey towards improved hearing clarity and cognitive health.

QUESTION #6

What if I still have questions after the initial consultation?

The initial consultation can be overwhelming for some people and for their family members—and can sometimes stretch to sixty minutes or more. In these situations, it can be difficult to ask every question, to process everything that is being said, and to understand the enormity of the diagnosis of hearing loss. Every patient of mine has my e-mail and phone number on my business card. I believe in an open discussion and dialogue and that many patients, and perhaps their family members, will have questions that come up even after the appointment is over.

I always invite and encourage patients to bring family and loved ones to their appointments. Bring a spouse, bring a child, bring a grandchild—it's okay because your hearing loss impacts every one of these people.

It is important that the patient and his or her loved ones understand exactly what is happening with the patient, exactly what the degree of hearing loss is, how the disorder can impact his or her life, how it can impact his or her cognitive function, and how it can impact his or her risk of developing dementia, which often leads to loss of independence and even institutionalization. At the initial consultation, there will also be a medical recommendation presented for how to treat the hearing loss. There is no one-size-fits-all treatment plan. NeuroTechnology™ offers a wide array of options that are often dictated by the test results and patients' needs.

QUESTION #7

When is the best time to treat my hearing loss?

A.S.A.P. Hearing loss is associated with increased rates of diabetes, heart disease, kidney disease, thyroid disease, problems with balance, falling, and the development of dementia.

The longer you wait, the more you are depriving the brain of proper auditory stimulation, often referred to as auditory deprivation. Your brain is not getting the proper auditory stimulation and auditory cues that it needs to run at 100%. The brain is a very simple "Use it or Lose It" mechanism, and auditory input can help to provide the proper, constant stimulation our brains are accustomed to and designed to receive. Hearing is not a sense to take for granted. Yet the statistics are alarming—it is estimated that only 20% of individuals with hearing loss actually seek medical treatment. Without the proper treatment of hearing loss, the brain is being asked to work on overload, constantly.

In neuroscience, we call this "Cognitive Overload"—asking the brain to process auditory, visual, and other cues just to put together a simple sentence.

Consider this sentence:

> *Hi, Martha! How is your puppy doing? Is he eating and growing okay? I hope we can get our dogs together soon to play.*

If we filter this sentence through a typical mild age-related hearing loss with compromised clarity (e.g., difficulty with consonant discrimination), the sentence could be perceived as this:

> *i, Mara! ow i our uy oing? I e eaing and groing o? I oe e an ge our do ogeer oon o ay.*

I think you will agree that this is rather alarming. Remember earlier when we discussed patients with mild hearing loss missing 50-60% of words at near-normal conversational volume? This is what it could sound like to the patient with auditory-only cues. Of course, the brain will use visual cues, lip-reading, etc. to fill in the missing pieces—but the brain was not designed to take on that much stress and effort just to understand a simple sentence.

This cognitive overload is hypothesized to be one of the leading reasons that individuals with hearing loss can be FIVE TIMES more likely to develop dementia.

QUESTION #8

What if I am nervous about treating my hearing loss?

Undergoing treatment for any medical disorder can be overwhelming to patients and to their family members. Fortunately, today's NeuroTechnology™ has alleviated most of the worries and concerns about treating hearing loss. The technology is specifically designed to be discretely worn all day and fit comfortably in the patient's ear. With enhanced clarity features, background noise cancellation filters, and wireless connectivity, today's hearing loss treatment options are simple and sometimes even fun—you can connect your NeuroTechnology™ to all sorts of home electronics including light bulbs, coffee pots, doorbells, etc.—but this is beyond the scope of this book!

QUESTION #9

Why can't we wait until next year to treat my hearing loss?

Hearing loss, for some reason, seems to be the perfect thing for patients to try and put off "until next year." Patients will try to rationalize their hearing loss: "Oh, this is normal for my age" or "Everybody mumbles." If patients don't understand the unintended consequences of waiting to treat hearing loss and the medical conditions associated with hearing loss, how can they be expected to understand the importance of starting treatment of hearing loss today!

Simply stated, the organ of hearing (i.e., the cochlea) has a finite amount of receptor cells—referred to as hair cells. These are not like the hair on your head. They are microscopic filament-like fibers you might remember from looking at a paramecium in high school biology. Remember those?? There are thousands of these hair cells in the cochlea and they are akin to the rods and cones of the eye, which receive stimulation and pass along the information as a complex series of neurochemical signals to the brain. Some hearing losses are age-related, depending on your genetics. This problem is becoming more prominent in our society as we live longer, more active and engaged lives. Other factors that affect the health of the inner ear are poor blood oxygenation (found in conditions like heart disease, diabetes etc), noise exposure, head trauma and viral/bacterial infections.

With this progressive degenerative disorder, there is a gradual, continual loss of hair cells within the cochlea. These cells each have multiple nerve fibers responsible for relaying information to the brain to process sounds and conversation. As each cell dies with age and excessive exposure to noise (compounded by the combination of the two), the cells will die and so, too, will the attached neurons.

A recent study from Johns Hopkins found significant cerebral atrophy (AKA brain shrinkage) in the brains of individuals with hearing loss —likely the result of the progressive degenerative nature of hearing loss. The cerebral atrophy found in these individuals is reminiscent of the global cerebral atrophy observed in individuals with dementia.

Treating hearing loss early has many advantages—predicated on "Use It or (Continue to) Lose It." Treating hearing loss cannot prevent further damage caused by our genetics or prior exposure to loud noise but it can help maintain clarity and fine resolution of speech understanding as the disorder progresses. Numerous studies have been done over the years to understand the impact of only using one hearing aid when the patient had equal amounts of hearing loss in both ears. The results are definitive. Two ears are better than one.

The untreated ear's ability to perform word discrimination tasks are significantly reduced compared to the treated ear. Looking back on these results, they almost seem like common sense—the brain was designed to receive input from two ears and can respond adversely if only stimulated by one. I often joke with my patients who ask, "Do I have to treat both ears?" by asking them "If you needed glasses, would you wear a monocle like the Monopoly-man?!" In all seriousness, the importance of treating hearing loss early cannot be understated. Maintaining the strength and vitality of neural connections of the ear to the brain is key to the successful treatment of hearing loss.

PART 3

FOCUSING ON A PLAN THAT WORKS FOR YOU

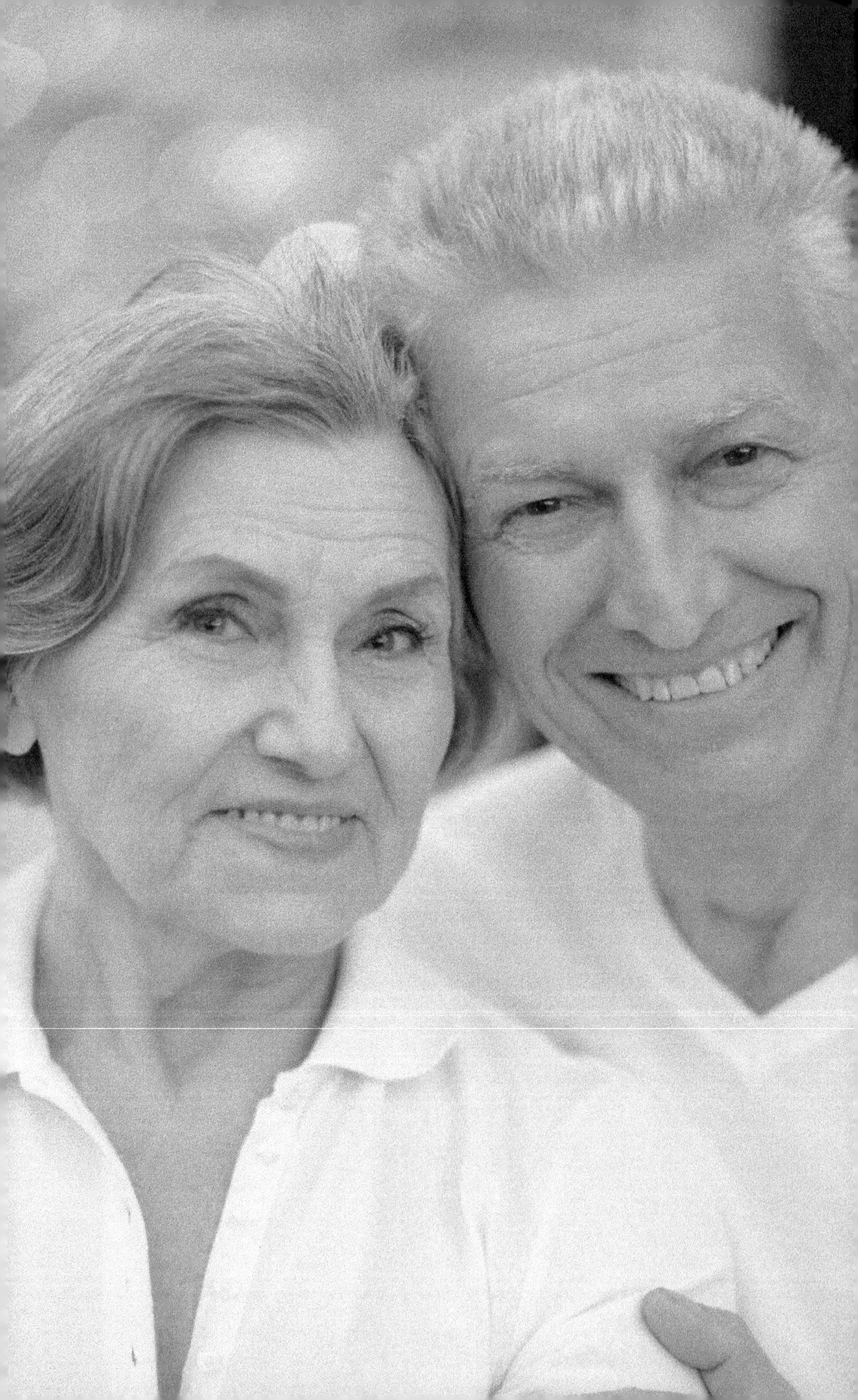

Is there an ideal patient?

The ideal patient is a person who understands both the medical and personal consequences of untreated hearing loss. A person who understands that their hearing loss is not just about them but understands that hearing loss impacts their entire family, their group of friends, and their community. An ideal patient is somebody who is daily invested in their life, somebody who is invested in active aging, somebody who is invested in living independently, somebody who wants to stay engaged and who wants to be a part of the conversation, somebody who wants to be a part of their family and who wants to remain engaged in their community.

The ideal patient has to accept the cost-benefit ratio when it comes to treating hearing loss; and I hope that this book has helped patients understand that it's nearly impossible to put a dollar value on improved health. I believe the ideal patient truly wants to stay involved, wants to grow, wants to remain independent, and wants to make the most of every day and every relationship that he or she has. That is an ideal patient. If you are, or know someone that fits this description, please help them begin treatment of their hearing loss as soon as possible. You are always welcome at my clinic or at one of the Audigy member-clinics in your area.

I suppose on the other side of the coin is the "not ideal patient"—the person whose wife, child, or grandchild dragging them into the office, and the patient is there just to get them to stop bugging them. That's not an ideal patient, although we have helped motivate many of them to realize what they need to do for themselves and their families. This type of patient must realize that there is a problem and they must want to make a change. As you know, "you can lead a horse to water, but you can't make it drink."

QUESTION #10

What treatment options are available to me when I'm ready to start treating my hearing loss?

I get this question often as I meet new patients, and even from family and friends. My answer is always the same: **NeuroTechnology™**. Advances in technology specifically designed to treat the cognitive aspects of hearing loss, not just make things louder, have significantly improved patient care and patient satisfaction.

But my next response is always "*You must see an Audigy member-clinic to determine which form of NeuroTechnology™ suits you and your hearing loss best.*"

While the most important factor in determining treatment is always based on the patient's hearing profile and health care history, specific options can be based on several factors including: addressing specific patient symptoms (difficulty in certain acoustic environments, tinnitus, etc.), dexterity (can the patient manipulate an invisible hearing device?), and personal preferences (color, size, etc.,). Your hearing health care provider can help you understand which form of NeuroTechnology™, what shape and size, and which specific features can help you hear your best and keep you engaged in conversation.

QUESTION #11

What treatment options are available for the ringing in my ears (aka tinnitus)?

As a clinical audiologist, one of the most common questions, and complaints, I get from my patients is about the 'ringing' in their ears! Tinnitus (pronounced either TIH˙nih˙ tus or tuh˙NYE˙ tus) is defined as a sensation of sound in your ears, sometimes in your head. Each person with tinnitus has a different sound experience; for most it is described as a "ringing" sound, but many patients also report a shooshing, buzzing, or whooshing sound—similar to the sounds inside a conch shell.

I have tinnitus. In January of 2005, while driving my son to a school function, I was hit head on by a drunk driver. The impact caused my airbags to deploy (which is like a gunshot going off at close range). My son thankfully was uninjured. I, however, sustained major facial bruising, damaged tendons in my right hand and permanent damage to my inner ears (greater on the left side, as the sound wave from the exploding airbag bounced off of the driver's side window and then to my left ear. This experience has certainly made me empathetic to anyone who suffers from tinnitus. Imagine a loud ringing sound that you just cannot get away from, day or night, regardless of how loud sound is around you. Tinnitus is responsible for many sleep deprived nights. Because of this experience, I have researched, learned, and personally experienced many of the options for tinnitus treatment that are available today. I am currently evaluating a wristband that uses cognitive retraining that has been shown to reduce the perception of tinnitus. I routinely use a sound application on an iPod that allows me to listen to an audiobook to fall asleep at night. I take specific vitamins that have helped reduce to severity of my tinnitus. I wear NeuroTechnology in both ears that helps my brain be less aware of the ringing. I am always on the lookout for treatments that can be a help to me and my patients.

It is currently estimated that nearly 50,000,000 American adults live with tinnitus. Tinnitus is experienced by approximately 80% of people living with hearing loss.

Too many people dismiss the ringing, when in fact this sound essentially represents an internal alarm alerting you that something is not as it should be. Whether the tinnitus is constant, only noticeable in a quiet room or at night, pulsating or seems to have certain triggers (i.e., exercise or caffeine), it is important that the root cause of the problem be determined, and a proper treatment plan be put in place with your hearing health care specialist. In some people, the tinnitus can interfere with daily life and result in depression, anxiety and affect concentration.

What is the cause of tinnitus?

The most common cause of tinnitus is damage to the sensory organ of hearing, the cochlea (i.e., the inner ear). The cochlea is to hearing what your eyes are to vision. Within the cochlea are those tiny filament-like cells called hair cells. When these cells are damaged, the nerves that connect the hair cells to the brain (and give us the ability to hear), become permanently damaged; and often times the ringing will ensue.

How Do the Sensory Cells In My Ear Get Damaged?

The sensory cells in the ear are most vulnerable to aging. Think about it—as we get older, we tend not to see as well or see as sharply as we used to, especially in low-light environments. Unfortunately, the same process can happen in our ears as we age; we tend not to hear as clearly, especially in noisy situations.

Another common cause of tinnitus is excessive noise exposure, either a single intense noise (like a shotgun blast or an airbag) or long-term exposure either from work or play (e.g., musicians, concert attendees, carpenters, machinists, landscapers, etc.).

But Why Do My Ears Ring?

Tinnitus is most often the result of a "Central Gain" in neural activity that occurs when there is a loss of proper neural stimulation from the ear to the brain. More simply, when the brain is not stimulated in the case of individuals with hearing loss (even a mild hearing loss), the brain will increase activity to make up for the missing input.

This "Central Gain" is neurologically analogous to "Phantom Limb" phenomenon studied in neuroscience. In cases where damage occurs to the peripheral nervous system—such as when a solider loses a limb in battle—the central nervous system (aka the brain) will undergo adaptive changes that can often result in the perception of pain. Our ear's perception of pain is the ringing. Based on my experience of the sudden damage to my ear, my theory is that the damaged hair cells are sending incorrect chemical and electrical signals to my brain that is interpreted as sound in the absence of a true auditory stimulus.

Treatment For Your Tinnitus

Unfortunately, too many patients have said to me, "I have tinnitus, and I've been told there is nothing that I can do about it." I emphatically say to each of these patients—that is not true, because my tinnitus is not nearly as loud or obtrusive as it used to be. Is there a cure for tinnitus? No. Are there proven FDA-approved treatment options available to reduce, and in some cases, eliminate, the ringing? YES!

The single most effective treatment option available for patients suffering with tinnitus is NeuroTechnology™. The FDA (Food and Drug Administration) has approved treatment for individuals with tinnitus by providing the brain with restored proper stimulation. And while most people with tinnitus also suffer with hearing loss, that is not always the case. Fortunately, newly available NeuroTechnology™ has been designed for people with hearing loss and for individuals with (so called) "normal" hearing. Many studies show that patients who use the tinnitus support technology note a significant reduction in their daily tinnitus experience—with some even reporting that "the ringing is gone all day".

QUESTION #12

What if I have "total hearing loss" in one of my ears? (And what is a CROS System?)

As a general rule of thumb, hearing ability in the two ears should be near equal to each other. After all, your ears are the same age. If you have a history of noise exposure it was likely the same in both ears, and if you were prescribed a medicine with a side-effect that could impact hearing, it will impact both ears similarly.

But, in some patients, hearing in one ear will be much worse than the other. This can result from a host of otologic issues, including viral infection of the ear, physical trauma to the ear, and of unknown origin (medically diagnosed as "idiopathic hearing loss") which is a funny sounding medical diagnosis. It doesn't mean that your doctors are idiots! According to the Merriam Webster dictionary, "idiopathic" means "arising spontaneously or from an obscure or unknown cause".

The separation of hearing levels between the two ears can sometimes be dramatic or even complete. Unfortunately, some patients have a "dead ear" (medically defined as anacusis) with normal hearing in the other ear. In other patients, there is an "asymmetric hearing loss" which implies hearing loss in one ear and even worse hearing in the other ear. The brain was designed to hear with two ears, and it will function best with equal hearing in both ears. Binaural (two-ear) hearing has significant benefits that include increased sound localization ability (e.g., figuring out where sound is coming from in the room) and enhanced perception of speech in noisy situations. These characteristics of binaural hearing are often referred to as the "Binaural Advantage." If you know somebody with "lopsided" hearing loss, you will notice that they always strategize to improve the listening environment by having the speaker(s) on their better hearing side.

While the course of treatment for individuals with significantly poorer hearing in one ear is different than the patient with symmetrical hearing loss, NeuroTechnology™ can be used to significantly enhance hearing and understanding in all listening situations.

Briefly, the most common NeuroTechnology™ used in these cases is referred to as a CROS System. CROS (Contralateral Routing of Signal) will take sound from the "dead" / worse side and route it over to the better side (even if there is some hearing loss in the "better" side). Using this technology allows the patient to access sound on the (otherwise) muted side of the body. While this patient may never perform as well as an individual treating equal levels of hearing loss in both ears, restoring perception of sound from the muted side of the body can offer significant relief in almost all listening situations.

QUESTION #13

Do they still make traditional hearing aids?

Yes, traditional hearing aids are still made. Mostly this traditional technology has been relabeled and is now masquerading as "new" over-the-counter (OTC) technology or personal sound amplification devices (PSAPs). Unfortunately, because the words "hearing aid" are very general and very common, it can be quite confusing for the patient. As I explain to my patients nearly every day:

> *"Your father (or grandfather) wore traditional hearing aids (and he probably hated them). This older technology was intended to make sounds louder regardless of location in the room, regardless of the volume of the incoming sounds, and regardless of what the patient did or didn't actually want to hear."*

As an audiologist seeing patients early on in my career, I was very disappointed by the limitations of the traditional hearing aid technology, but it was all that we had at the time. Things have certainly changed for the better!

QUESTION #14

So, what's the deal with new hearing aids and NeuroTechnology™?

(Most) new "hearing aids" are NeuroTechnology™.

In the last 10 years or so, there have been giant leaps and bounds in hearing aids towards improving listening experience for the patient (and thus increasing patient satisfaction). Prior to that time, the average patient satisfaction rating for traditional hearing aid experience was hovering around 70% to75% (as measured by the MarkeTrak survey).

If you now fast forward another ten years to present time, the most recent MarkeTrak survey examining patient satisfaction with hearing loss treatment has shown ***an improvement to 91%!*** I believe this number speaks for itself.

Treatment of hearing loss with traditional hearing aids is (thankfully) beginning to be phased out and replaced with NeuroTechnology™ designed to enhance hearing in all listening situations, enhance clarity of speech details, automatically provide an increased boost of volume for soft speakers, stimulate the brain, and increase cognitive function.

QUESTION #15

Is there such a thing as an invisible hearing aid?

Modern NeuroTechnology hearing aids are really hard to see on most patients. Like Wonder Woman's invisible jet plane—you can't see it, but it really cool! I get questions about this all the time from patients: "What is an invisible hearing aid?" and "Will my friends be able to see it?

When treating hearing loss with NeuroTechnology™, I have two principles that I always follow:

1. Use the right NeuroTechnology™ to treat the patient's hearing loss and improve cognitive health.

2. Respect the patient's desire for NeuroTechnology™ that is physically and aesthetically comfortable for them.

BUT… Principle #2 can never override Principle #1.

As a general rule of thumb in the tech world, the size of technology decreases over time. NeuroTechnology™ uses smaller, more powerful digital technology and processing to automatically adapt to the user's surroundings. I have always believed that treating hearing loss should require minimal effort from the patient. The hearing-impaired person needs to start using NeuroTechnology™ when he or she wakes up in the morning and then simply remove it before falling asleep—and do nothing in between! NeuroTechnology™ has ushered in the age of effortless hearing loss treatment.

Advances in design and technology allow for the user to be hands free—no more buttons for environment (i.e., push the button twice when in a noisy restaurant, push three times when in the gym, push the button four times when on the phone, etc.) and no more spin-wheels to adjust the volume up and down. Innovations in NeuroTechnology™ allow for automatic adaptation to dynamic environmental listening situations (e.g., listening to speech as you go from a quiet room to a noisy room), and it can automatically adapt to incoming volume to maintain the normal fluctuations in the volume of voices and background noise. The most advanced feature of NeuroTechnology™ is noise cancellation that delivers increased access to clear speech in noisy listening situations (more on this in the bonus question!).

While NeuroTechnology™ is the circuitry inside the device, the device can come in different shapes and sizes to best fit your hearing loss and your ear.

NeuroTechnology™ Options for Treating Hearing Loss

Invisible Treatment Options

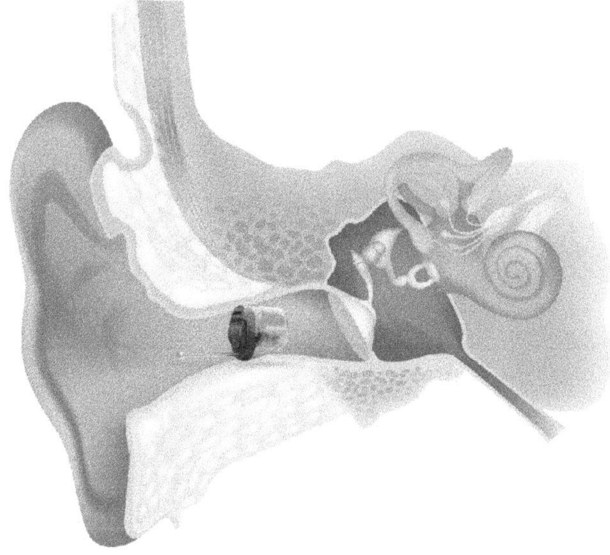

Invisible technology is seated comfortably in the ear canal for all day comfort and maximum discreteness.

Once placed in your ear, this technology is hassle-free—you may even forget you're wearing the device! And that's the point. Hearing loss shouldn't hold you back, and neither should your hearing solution. Features in today's invisible technology options include:

- An invisible and custom fit. Some devices can be deeply fit inside your ear canal with personal customization for all day comfort.

- Low battery reminders. Devices can remind you in your ear, your phone (if compatible) by text, or email that your batteries (or your loved ones batteries) are low, and as of this writing, deeply fit completely in the canal devices only use replaceable batteries, not rechargeable ones.
- Easy adaptation to new sounds with automatic volume control and adaptation to the listening environment.
- Sound comfort technology designed to provide distortion-free listening comfort for loud sounds while ensuring ultimate clarity.

Mini "Receiver in the Ear" Options

Groundbreaking NeuroTechnology™ is fast and precise enough to analyze and follow the dynamics of the entire auditory environment and differentiate between speech and background noise. Briefly (and without getting too lost in technical details), NeuroTechnology™ is capable of sampling sounds in the environment 100 times per second to decide on how to optimally perform and restore clarity; whereas traditional hearing aids were barely capable of analyzing the sound environment and capped out at a sampling rate of less than 5 times per second.

Advances in miniaturization of technology have led to the breakthrough of new NeuroTechnology™ found to support brain function, including working memory, selective attention, and processing speed (see Bibliography section for report from Dr. Desjardin, University of Texas, El Paso). These new devices have three features designed specifically to maintain the brain's innate ability to hear in all different listening situations:

- **Clearer Hearing in Background Noise.** By separating important speech from background noise by as much as 10 decibels, this new technology provides 30% better speech understanding and clarity in noise.
- **Enhanced Clarity = Enhanced Memory Recall.** Individuals with hearing loss can have difficulty with working memory, thought to be the result of distorted auditory input to the brain. NeuroTechnology™ can provide 20% more capacity to recall and remember words* by increasing the clarity of the signal being processed by the brain.

- **Reduced Mental Effort.** Many patients describe hearing loss as being "exhausting." Normal hearing is relatively effortless in most listening situations. But to an individual with hearing loss, even a simple conversation at work with a colleague or while out fishing with the grandchildren can require major effort and use of all available mental resources, including lip-reading. NeuroTechnology can offer the hearing-impaired user relief by reducing the "cognitive load" (e.g., mental effort) by 20%*; making the conversation significantly easier to follow in all situations.

Other features include:

- Hands-free wireless surround sound hearing on compatible smart phone.
- Rechargeable batteries. No more batteries going dead at inconvenient moments. No more batteries dropped on the floor. No more unexpectedly running out of batteries at a critical moment. The devices are recharged nightly by putting them into a special charging case and can last up to 18 hours on a single charge.
- Wireless compatibility with any TV to enhance the clarity of the signal. A separate accessory may be required.
- Control of your internet connected devices at home, including the thermostat, lights, and even certain cooking appliances.

Let's join in with all current NeuroTechnology™ users and celebrate!

Gone are the days of clunky "beige banana" hearing aids for all but the most severe of hearing losses!

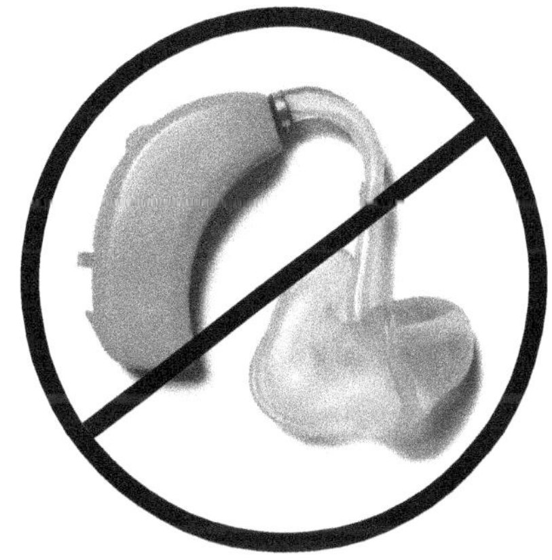

QUESTION #16

Are Over-the-Counter Hearing Aids Right for Me?

For persons with a diagnosed mild hearing loss, an OTC device might be the perfect solution. What does a "mild hearing loss" mean? If a person is missing 25-30% of the sounds in a normal listening environment with a person speaking at an average volume, that person has a mild hearing loss. This person probably has issues only in certain situations and the hearing loss is having a mild impact on their listening functions. They would most likely use their OTC device on a part-time basis. Because of the minimal impact and the part-time use, this person would not be considered a good candidate for prescriptive amplification. It's kind of like reading glasses. You don't need to wear them full-time and you get them at the drugstore.

Over the counter hearing devices have a potential for helping many people with mild hearing loss.

The Over the Counter (OTC) Hearing Aid Act was passed as part of the 115th United States Congress in 2017. This law required the food and drug administration (FDA) to propose a rule that would establish an OTC hearing aid category for adults with perceived mild to moderate hearing loss within three years of passage of the legislation. Due to a combination of factors (the slow process of legislation in general, combined with the Covid pandemic) this rule was finalized in October 2022.

History of Electronic Hearing Aids.

Hearing aid manufacturers have been around since the early 1900s. The first vacuum tube hearing aid was patented in 1920. These are companies with years of research and development with deep understanding of how humans hear and process sound, especially those with impaired hearing. Making all sound louder is not what helps people with impaired hearing. Prescriptive devices are programmed for an individuals hearing loss, their particular ear characteristics, their particular hearing lifestyle and their individual preferences.

As early as the 1980s mail order hearing aids were available for purchase. These devices were often simple amplifiers people could order through the mail. Fast forward to the Internet. For many years it has been possible to buy some type of amplification device online. These devices were typically simple amplifiers, were made in China, and were pretty clunky looking. They could also be found in the "as seen on TV" aisle in your local drugstore.

As of this writing, OTC hearing aids are being manufactured by electronics companies, not hearing aid manufacturers. That may change with time. Hearing aid manufacturers must adhere to manufacturing rules for medical devices that electronics companies do not.

The concept of OTCs was welcomed by the audiology community to help people with diagnosed mild hearing loss. The intention was to have a solution be available for people who needed hearing help only in some situations and were designed to be used part-time. Prescriptive devices are designed to be worn during all waking hours for people who need hearing help in most or all situations. Professionals in the audiology world (including myself) have long petitioned manufacturers of hearing aids to make an inexpensive device that could be used by people who have mild hearing loss and needed only part-time help. I've seen thousands of this type of person over the years and did not have anything that was appropriate for them.

Throughout my career the model of hearing care has been pretty straightforward. A person or their family would notice their loved one was not hearing/understanding. Some would go straight to an audiologist or maybe even go to a "free hearing test" place to get checked out. Others would inform their doctor of their symptoms with hearing and they would be referred to a medical professional (typically an audiologist) for evaluation. Once evaluated, a plan of care would be put into place. That plan of care could cover anything from earwax removal, back to their primary care for treatment, to a referral to an ENT, to a recommendation for tinnitus treatment, to a recommendation for a recheck after treatment, to a recommendation for preferential seating in a classroom, to a recommendation of hearing aid use. If a medical problem was found, the patient was sent for medical or surgical treatment.

It has been my experience as an audiologist most people are typically very unaware of their hearing. Hearing loss is typically very gradual over many years. Because of the gradual onset, the brain is tuned to listening through their hearing loss and considers that input “normal”. Because they are experiencing that filter through their hearing loss, they are typically missing some of the sounds of speech, so it sounds like people are mumbling. By the time most people are seen by an audiologist it is because their family members are growing increasingly frustrated trying to communicate with them. I have frequently heard the following statement. “My hearing is fine. People just mumble. If they would talk right, I would hear just fine”.

I have seen patients that think they hear “just fine” have results that show a moderate to severe hearing loss. Everyone has a different hearing profile. Some people hear low pitches better than others. Some are missing middle pitches or have different loudness growth than someone else. Many complain of “not understanding” rather than hearing. Most people with mild hearing loss may not even be aware that they have a hearing loss. Hearing loss is a symptom. Symptoms must be addressed.

A few years ago I rechecked a patient’s hearing that had been wearing hearing aids for years and found her hearing had worsened greater than expected. I had her go to her primary care doctor to be checked out. It turned out her carotid arteries were 80-90% blocked and she needed surgery to prevent a stroke. The resulting loss of blood flow and oxygen to her brain and ears had caused further hearing loss. If she had not had a diagnostic hearing exam this issue would not have been found.

Most audiologists don’t have a problem with the idea of over-the-counter devices for persons with mild hearing loss. What we do have a problem with is it requires self diagnosis, which raises the risk of medical issues not being found and addressed in time.

Somewhere along the line someone decided getting a hearing test was providing a “barrier to care”. Is getting your vision checked or your cholesterol checked a “barrier to care”? No, they are not. Just like other medical testing, hearing exams are covered by insurance and typically take 45 minutes to an hour of time. That small investment of time is well worth it when the big picture of a person’s health is considered. Self diagnosis is rarely a good idea when there is some type of problem a person is having that relates to their health.

Once an exam and communication interview is completed, your Doctor of Audiology will make recommendations for a plan of care. If it is determined there are no medical issues that require treatment and a hearing loss is found, then recommendations will be made that fit your particular hearing and communication needs. In my experience, people who are missing 25 to 35% of the sounds that exist in normally spoken speech need only part-time help or situational help. These issues could be covered by OTC device, bluetooth headphones that are synced to your television or computer, or just counseling regarding management of environments, the importance of room acoustics and use of visual cues.

Prescriptive devices are recommended for those patients who are missing 35-40% or greater of the sounds in normal conversational speech. Those patients typically are more aggravated by their issues with their hearing (or their family is aggravated) and are in need of a full time solution that is customized to their particular needs. Prescriptive devices include a treatment plan that covers all services, repairs, office visits, earwax removal, etc for a period of time. The standard treatment plan at my office covers the above for 3 years.

When an audiologist fits a hearing aid, objective measurements are made to determine what the hearing aid is doing at different pitches and different presentation levels to tune the hearing aid specifically to your individual ear and your individual hearing loss. This ensures sounds are at the correct level to be heard but not so loud they can injure your hearing. Without these measurements, it is impossible to know if the amplification device has been set optimally for you. OTC devices are not assessed in this way as the settings are based only on what a person with impaired hearing is deciding what might sound better to them.

On the first day of hearing aid fitting, most patients indicate sounds don't seem normal to them which is because the brain is not used to hearing many of these softer sounds. It may take several weeks of full-time use (all waking hours) to adjust to a new hearing aid fitting because the brain must adapt to this new normal. Prescriptive devices are adjusted gradually to maximize benefit and comfort. Having a professional (your audiologist) coaching a patient through this process has been shown to have better results over time. It is also important to understand that hearing loss is a problem that requires ongoing care. Hearing must be monitored over time and when hearing aids are part of a treatment plan, they must be cleaned, updated, and checked on a regular basis. When working with a Doctor of Audiology, your treatment plan is part of the fitting process.

PART 4

FINANCING YOUR HEARING LOSS TREATMENT WITHOUT BREAKING THE BANK

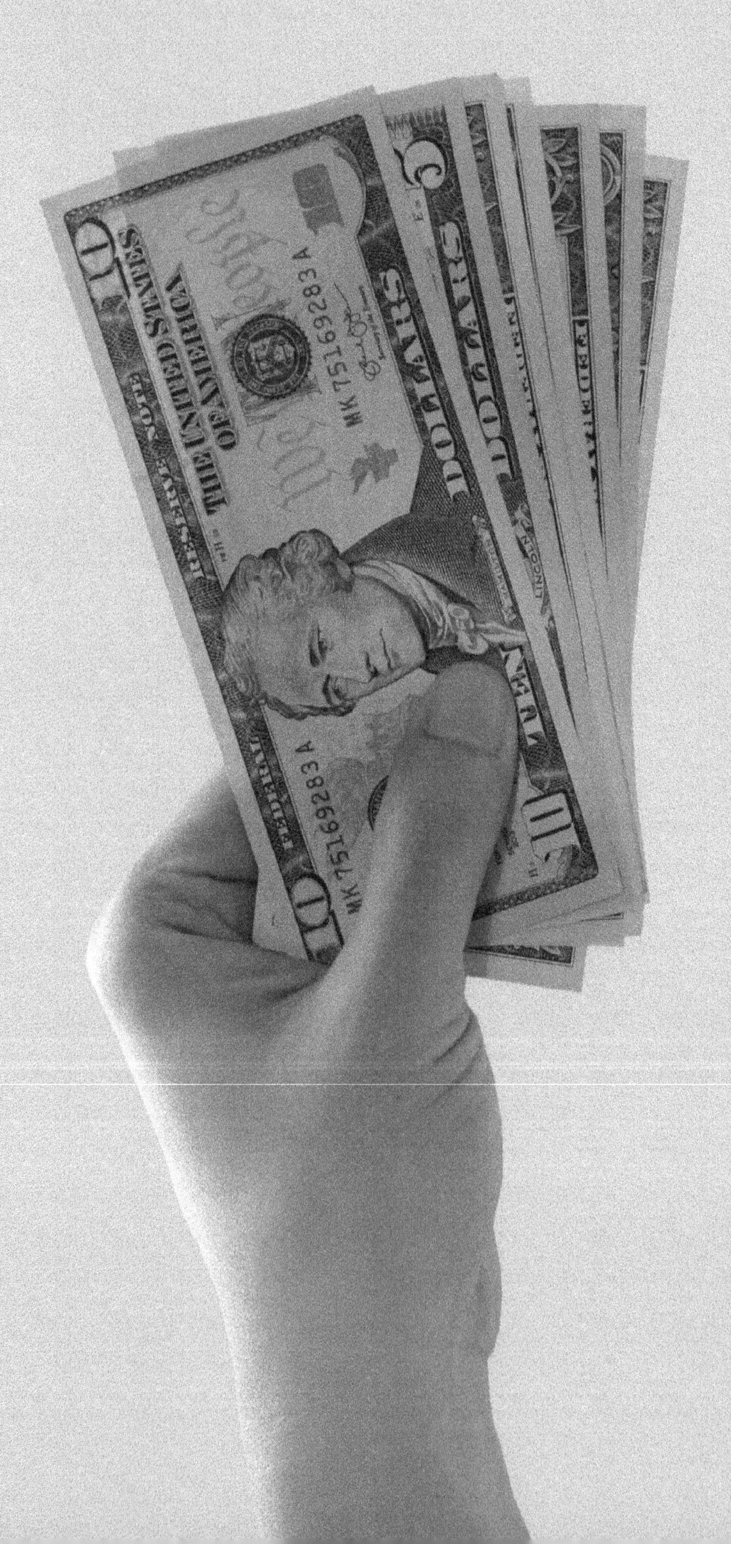
THE UNITED STATES OF AMERICA
FEDERAL RESERVE NOTE
MK75169283A
DOLLARS
TEN
10

QUESTION #17

How much will my "new ears" cost me?

Answer: It depends.

Throughout this book I have alluded to NeuroTechnology™ treatment options as the "gold standard" of treating hearing loss. Specific recommendations will rely on a number of factors (e.g., degree of hearing loss, symptoms, amount of time living with untreated hearing loss, etc.). However, with that said, I have over twenty years of horror stories of patients trying to "save a buck." I know patients who have thrown away $30, $300, even as much as $3,000 on a "sound machine in their ear" that amplifies volume. Some have tried traditional hearing aids that only make sounds louder; some have tried online or over-the-counter (OTC) devices; some have tried Personal Sound Amplifiers (PSAPs); some have even tried "mail-order" hearing aids. Regardless, each time these patients come back asking for something that actually works! I take no issue with patients trying to save money and make good economic decisions, but even with health care…you get what you pay for. Treating the progressive degenerative nature of age-related hearing loss is no different than treating other major medical disorders as you age. As an example, imagine yourself, or a loved one, in a situation where hip-replacement surgery is required. Could you imagine your surgeon asking the following question?

> *"Would you like me to replace your hip and restore 30%, 70%, or maximum percent mobility?"*

Here is another example, imagine saying to your heart surgeon, after he/she lets you know that you are required to undergo triple by-pass and heart valve replacement:

> *"Doc, if you don't mind, I'm going to shop on Amazon for a replacement valve to try and save a few bucks...even if it doesn't pump the adequate amount of blood to keep my body oxygenated and healthy."*

While both of these scenarios may seem far-fetched and ridiculous, unfortunately the retail aspect of hearing health care has "poisoned the well" for too many people living with hearing loss and has made treating hearing loss a very confusing, onerous process for the patient.

We trust all of our health care providers to use their knowledge and experience to provide us with the best, most medically sound treatment recommendation, regardless of price. You should expect the same from your doctor of audiology. If your clinician is reputable (e.g., is referred to by local physicians, has many five-star reviews on Google, has readily available current patient liaisons to speak with, etc.), is an Audigy member-clinic, and has longevity in the community, then you can rest assured that their pricing structure is standard and that the only variable is the cost of technology (pre-set by the manufacturer).

NeuroTechnology™ is the number one most effective, FDA (Food and Drug Administration) approved treatment for hearing loss and has the highest recorded level of patient satisfaction.

QUESTION #18

What is the cost of not treating my hearing loss?

Answer: Possibly a lot more than you think!

Throughout this book we have discussed the positive impact of treating hearing loss and the dire consequences of not treating hearing loss. It is difficult to assign a true monetary value to both of these scenarios, but I will give it my best shot!

Here are two examples.

1. Hearing loss can increase the risk of developing dementia by 200-500%. Treating hearing loss is reported as the single most effective modifiable factor to preventing dementia. Given these two medical research findings, it is not unreasonable to calculate the cost of treating a patient with dementia that could have possibly been avoided by treating his or her hearing loss at an earlier age. Statistics show that the average family will spend approximately $57,000.00 per year to cover health care costs and manage the care of a loved one with dementia.

2. Hearing loss increases the risk of falls in seniors. Treating hearing loss can significantly reduce the risk of falling. Again, given these two medical research findings, it is not unreasonable to calculate the cost of treating a patient who falls and compare it to the cost of treating hearing loss. Falling over the age of sixty-five is the #1 cause of injury related deaths. And once a person falls, he or she is two times more likely to fall again. The Center for Disease Control and Prevention (CDC) estimates that the average medical cost associated with a fall that results in hospitalization is over $30,000.00 (and the cost of treatment increases with age).

In addition to dementia and falls, co-morbidity of hearing loss (i.e., other diseases that are correlated with hearing loss) extends to diabetes, coronary disease, thyroid disease, and others.

QUESTION #19

How do I pay for my "new ears"?

Like any major medical procedure, audiology procedures can cost several thousand dollars, not all of which are covered by your insurance (depending on your plan!)

How much you will have to pay out of pocket depends on several factors, including the NeuroTechnology™ recommended, the procedures involved, and, of course, the specifics of your insurance policy. One way many of my patients pay for their treatment is by utilizing creative benefits. For example, using their Flexible Spending Account (FSA), financing at 0%, using tax returns, and even using the cost towards their medical expenses benefit on their tax returns (warning—I am not an accountant and do not even play one on TV— so always ask your accountant how to best proceed with all tax matters).

How to use Flexible Spending and eliminate the headache of using it!

Just to make sure we are all on the same page, "Flex Spending" is accessible through your work benefit package. It allows you to set aside a certain amount of money per year, TAX-FREE, to be used towards medical expenses. NeuroTechnology™ and treating hearing loss is a medical expense.

Step 1—Sign Up Early!

Perhaps you already follow the "5 P's to Success," (Proper Planning Prevents Poor Performance!) but in case you don't, this is one thing you want to plan early for so you can maximize the benefit. Many employees set higher limits than you think on the amount of Flexible Spending dollars you can contribute and access.

I have seen employees with as much as $2,500.00 and some with even $5,000.00 in Flex-Spending dollars available to them. Failure to sign up early could cost you more in out-of-pocket medical expenses, especially if your plan is not up and ready before you or a loved one needs to treat his or her hearing loss. If you have a new plan, work with your human resource contact to sign up early for next year in order to maximize your savings.

Step 2—Notify Your Employer of Family Status Change.

Different employers have different sign-up deadlines for the Flexible Spending plans, but typically at the beginning of the year your employer asks how much money you want to contribute for the year. The problem with making annual decisions about health care coverage is obvious—life happens and sometimes it's nearly impossible to plan ahead that far! You may apply for a Family Status Change for changes such as marriage, birth, divorce, or loss of a spouse's insurance. These are opportunities to add more coverage for hearing loss treatment expenses.

Step 3—Choose Wisely!

Finally, give some thought to calculating how much money to contribute to your flexible plan at work this year and every year. If you are considering hearing loss treatment for you or a family member, visit the specialist's office for an initial consultation.

Your patient care coordinator(s) can help you plan exactly how much money you should contribute to help reduce your out-of-pocket costs when it is time to pay for and receive your NeuroTechnology™.

Step 4—Use It or Lose It

Here's something you may not know (and frankly, has always puzzled me!) - if you put more money into your Flex Spending Account than you need or use, by law, you lose the money! Yikes!

BUT...you have three months after the end of the calendar year to submit claims for eligible medical expenses from the previous calendar year. Any money left in your account after this three-month period is forfeited.

To Finance or Not to Finance? 'Tis the Question!

As a human being with a family, home, and many other fiscal responsibilities, I understand the difference between things I need to buy and things I want to buy. Treating hearing loss is something that my patients need to invest in to ensure proper hearing and cognitive health. But not every patient is able to pay for treatment up front in a lump sum. A respectable specialist's office will be able to offer their patients the opportunity to finance. I can't provide the details of every office, or every offer, but these are the common financing options I have come across:

- 0% interest for as long as twelve to eighteen months.
- 12.9% interest with locked-in monthly payments for three to five years.
- Use of personal credit cards or credit unions which may have lower interest rates based on your own credit history.

QUESTION #20

Does my insurance cover the cost of NeuroTechnology™?

This is a loaded question—and one that I can only answer in general terms because health insurance coverage is a complex ever-changing set of rules, regulations, and specifics that make it impossible to make a blanket statement regarding your coverage.

After twenty years of patient care and working with nearly every flavor of insurance coverage, these are my two take-away messages:

1. Nearly every insurance plan, including Medicare, will cover the cost of the comprehensive hearing evaluation.
2. Many patients have some coverage for the cost of treatment (e.g., NeuroTechnology™).

I acknowledge that "nearly every" and "many" are vague terms, but this is the world of insurance we currently live in. I have worked with patients that have $100.00 of coverage and some with $10,000.00 in coverage (not that it should ever cost you that much!).

TIP: Do not be afraid to pick up the phone and ask your insurance company point blank: **"Do you cover the cost of treating hearing loss?"** Also, don't be afraid to call back and ask again (you would be shocked how many times our office has called insurance companies seeking this answer only to get a different answer each time we call!). At my office, our Patient Care Coordinators will work with the patient and their insurance company to maximize the patient's benefits and coverage.

BONUS SECTION

TREATING HEARING LOSS & YOUR OVERALL HEALTH

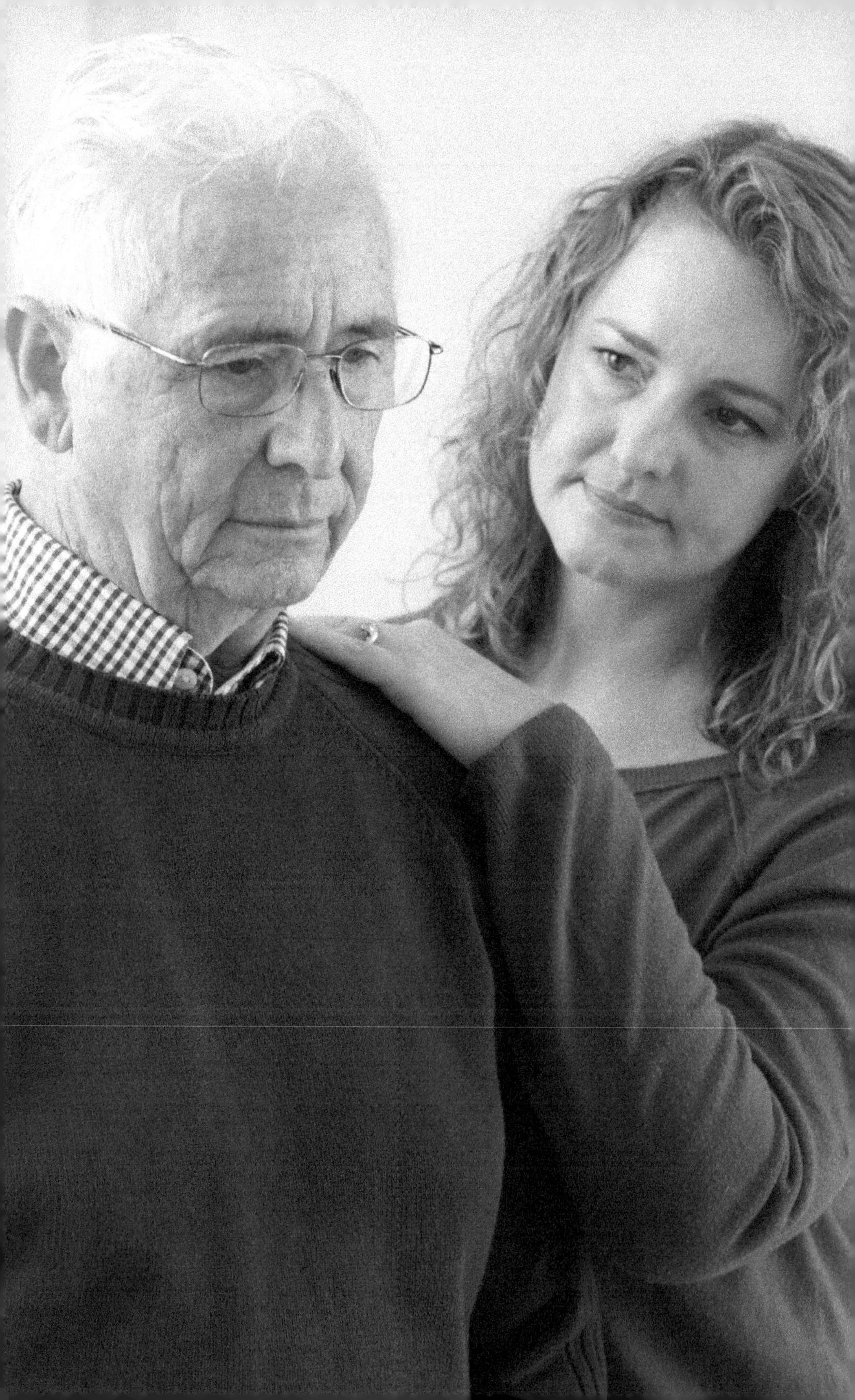

QUESTION #21

Has there been research into the relationship between hearing loss and dementia?

Age-related hearing loss is a progressive and degenerative disorder resulting from the loss of receptor cells (i.e., the hair cells) in the ear. Consequently, there is a significant reduction of the quantity and quality of neural connections from the ear to the brain. This slow-onset disorder can have a significant impact on several key brain areas, including the memory, hearing, speech, and language portions of cognitive function. Several key research studies have pointed to the potential links of hearing loss and dementia, including the groundbreaking work from Dr. Lin and his colleagues at Johns Hopkins Medical Center that indicate hearing loss can increase the risk of dementia by 200-500%.

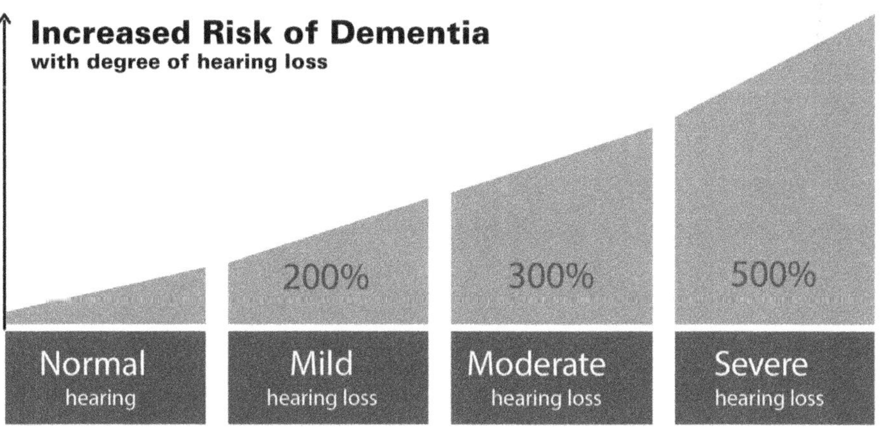

Summary data of relationship of hearing loss and increased risk of developing dementia.

The initial report first published in 2011 by scientists at Johns Hopkins Medical Center and the National Institute on Aging found that individuals with hearing loss (when compared to participants with normal hearing) are at a significantly higher risk of developing dementia as they age. The relationship of hearing loss and increased risk was rather simple: the more hearing loss they had, the higher the likelihood of developing the memory-robbing disease. "A lot of people ignore hearing loss because it's such a slow and insidious process as we age," Dr. Frank Lin (of Johns Hopkins Medical Center) says. "Even if people feel as if they are not affected, we're showing that it may well be a more serious problem."

Three risk factors associated with hearing loss and dementia include Social Isolation, Cerebral Atrophy and Cognitive Overload.

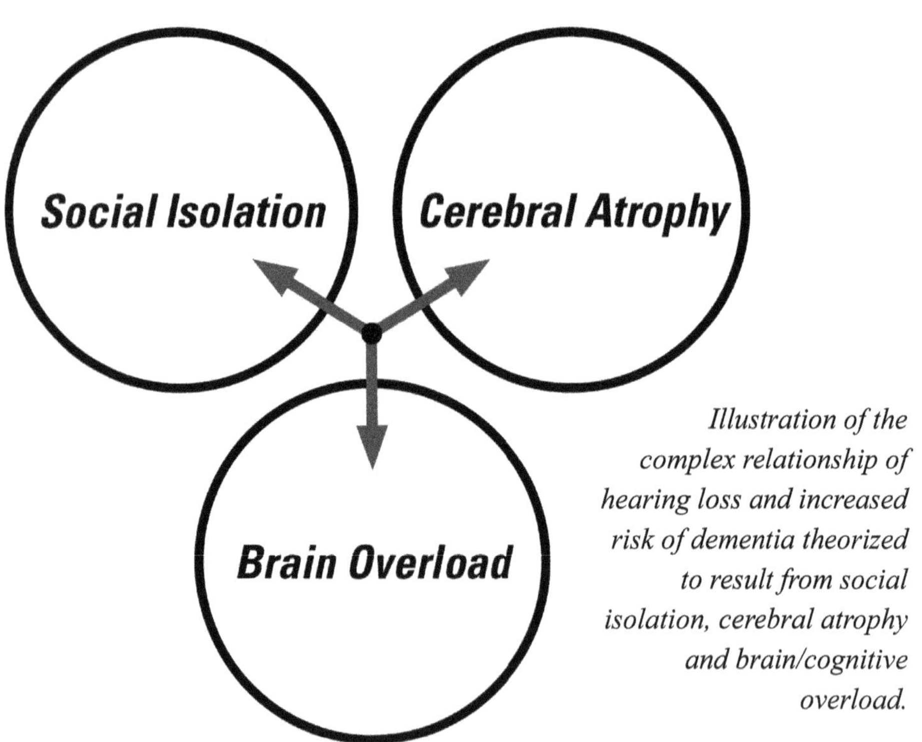

Illustration of the complex relationship of hearing loss and increased risk of dementia theorized to result from social isolation, cerebral atrophy and brain/cognitive overload.

Social Isolation

The impact of reduced social and physical activity.

Withdrawal from social situations is common in individuals with hearing loss. Many studies cite feelings of embarrassment, fear of making mistakes in conversations, and feeling like you are not part of the conversation as the common rational for individuals with hearing impairment to separate themselves from family, friends, and community. This retreat from social activity has even been found in individuals with a mild degree of hearing loss. In addition, individuals with hearing loss are less likely to engage in physical activity. Both increased social isolation and reduced physical activity are strong risk factors for the development of dementia.

"Blindness Separates You from Things,
Deafness Separates You from People".
— Helen Keller

Active Aging: How to Reduce Social Isolation

Active Aging—the process of optimizing opportunities for better health, continuing development of knowledge, and increased security in order to maximize quality of life as you age. The word "active" is used to describe a person's involvement with social, physical, economic, spiritual, and civic affairs. We all share the same goal to maintain autonomy and independence as we age, and thus we must rely on preserving the tenets of interdependence (socialization and reliance on family and loved ones) and intergenerational solidarity (maintaining companionship with age-matched peers) to insure active aging.

Both social isolation and depression are risk factors for the development of dementia, and both increase as we age. Being a lifelong learner and staying active is important to maintain a healthy, active brain, and can also reduce your risk of cognitive decline and dementia. Some studies have shown that social activities, larger social networks, and a history of social contact are associated with better cognitive function and reduced risk for cognitive decline.

Tips for active aging include:

- Sharing a meal with family and friends 3–5 times per week.
- Committing to an aerobics/exercise regimen.
- Learning a new hobby each year.
- Playing an instrument (or learning a new instrument).
- If you love to read…keep reading (and try to mix up the topics!).
- If you don't read much—try to read a book every other month.
- Participating in classes at your local senior center.
- Volunteering at a local hospital, shelter, etc.
- Going back to school. Many local state universities offer free tuition to people over 65.

Cerebral Atrophy (AKA Brain Shrinkage)

The association of a shrinking brain, resulting from the loss of neurons, with dementia has been long documented. Even people with MCI (Mild Cognitive Impairment) show signs of cerebral atrophy. In recent years, scientific studies using advanced brain imaging techniques (including fMRI -Functional Magnetic Resonance Imaging) have demonstrated that hearing impairment is associated with accelerated brain atrophy in both the overall brain, as well as even more advanced reductions in volume associated with the memory, hearing, speech, and language portions of the brain.

Individuals with hearing loss can experience significant cerebral atrophy. The most significant reduction in cerebral volume occurs in areas involved in memory, hearing, speech, and language.

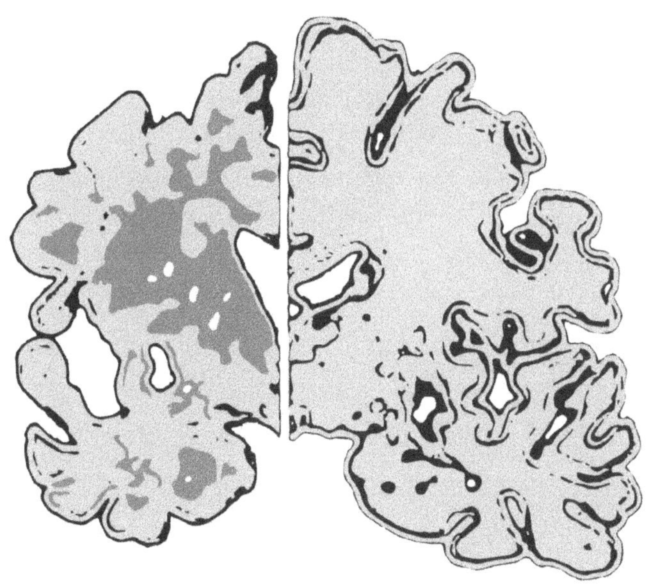

Schematic representing the potential cerebral atrophy in an individual with age-related hearing loss.

Cognitive Overload (i.e., Working Your Brain Too Hard in order Hear)

Hearing loss is not normal, and neither is the excessive strain that it can put on your brain. If you or somebody you love is experiencing hearing loss, you can observe this strain by watching the amount of effort required to follow a conversation. Patients will often joke and say, "I need to put my glasses on so I can hear you better." Requiring these extra visual and lip-reading cues may seem a natural way to fill in the missing speech details, but long term these coping mechanisms may have harmful effects on cognitive function.

With hearing loss, the brain is constantly on "overload" trying to fill in the missing pieces and follow the conversation. I often describe to my patients the taxing effect of hearing loss on brain function by describing the mental effort required to hear "is like driving 60 miles per hour in only second gear."

Increased cognitive load is considered a risk factor for developing dementia. Cognitive load, as measured by pupillometry (i.e., the size of the pupils indicates the amount of mental effort), can quantify how hard your brain is working to follow a conversation. Recent studies have found that individuals who treat their hearing loss do not work as hard to listen (i.e., have a reduced cognitive load) and have as much as a 20% increase in memory recall when following a conversation, even in noisy environments.

QUESTION #22

Can I reduce my increased risk of developing dementia by treating my hearing loss?

As I discuss the relationship of hearing loss and dementia with my patients, each seems to have the same follow up question for me: "Doc, if I treat my hearing loss, can I prevent or reduce my risk of developing dementia?" Thankfully, the data appears to be trending towards a resounding "Yes!" Recent reports have found a significant positive impact of treating hearing loss on cognitive health.

Treating Hearing Loss and the Impact on Cognitive Function

In a recent study investigating the relationship of treating hearing loss and cognitive function, it was found that current hearing loss treatments can improve brain function in people with hearing loss. It is understood that hearing loss, if left untreated, can lead to emotional and social consequences, reduced job performance, and diminished quality of life. Recently, studies have even shown that untreated hearing loss can interfere with cognitive abilities because so much mental effort is diverted toward understanding speech (i.e., cognitive overload).

The research was aimed at measuring core cognitive functions in subjects in their 50's and 60's beginning hearing loss treatment for the first time. After only two weeks of treatment, cognitive testing began to reveal a significant increase in scores for recalling words in working memory and selective attention tests, and that the processing speed for which participants selected the correct response was significantly faster. In summary: after only a couple of weeks, participants exhibited significant improvement in their cognitive function.

Treating Hearing Loss and the Impact on Risk of Developing Dementia

Since 2011, multiple long-term studies have provided strong evidence that treating hearing loss may eliminate the increased risk of developing dementia. **Dr. Lalwani at Columbia University noted that treating hearing loss...**

> *...may offer a simple, yet important, way to prevent or slow the development of dementia by keeping adults with hearing loss engaged in conversation and communication.*

Perhaps the most definitive report comes from the Lancet Commission, which presented a new life-course model documenting potentially modifiable risk factors for dementia. The Commission's report suggests that treating hearing loss is the **single most effective modifiable factor to preventing dementia**. Other modifiable factors include reducing depression, increasing physical activity, and reducing social isolation – each of which is positively impacted by treating hearing loss.

QUESTION #23

Can I really expect to be more socially active and engaged once I start treating my hearing loss?

Yes.

Throughout this book, I have been providing countless examples of how treating hearing loss can profoundly impact a patient's life and mental health. Frankly, connecting the dots of treating hearing loss to improvements in overall health and personal independence is simple. If you ask your primary care physician "doc, what do I need to do to be healthier?", the answer is guaranteed to include reduce stress, increase physical activity, stay socially active and engaged, lose weight, and eat healthy. Treating your hearing loss can help you achieve most of these goals. And achieving these goals is the key to healthy active aging. There are countless medical studies that find that people who do not treat hearing loss suffer from increased rates of depression, decreased socialization, and decreased physical activity. As an example, the National Council on Aging reported that individuals who do not treat hearing loss suffer from depression, anxiety, and decreased social activity. In contrast, individuals who proactively treat their hearing loss find improvements in relationships with family members (spouse, children, grandchildren, etc.), increases in feelings of self-esteem, and improvements in overall quality of life.

Connecting the Dots of Treating Hearing Loss and Improving Your Life

- Treating hearing loss can increase physical activity, reduce stress and anxiety, help with losing weight, and ultimately mean living a healthier and more independent lifestyle.

- Treating hearing loss can increase clarity of speech and the ability to follow conversation in background noise, increase socialization, help reduce the risk of depression, and ultimately mean living a healthier and more independent lifestyle.

- Treating hearing loss can increase auditory and environmental awareness, decrease the risk of falls, and ultimately mean living a healthier and more independent lifestyle.
- Treating hearing loss can increase cognitive function, can reduce the increased risk of developing dementia, and ultimately mean living a healthier and more independent lifestyle.

Hearing loss can be isolating for so many people for a multitude of reasons. But it doesn't have to be. If you've made it this far through the book, you have come to understand the importance of treating hearing loss and taking care of your brain—and how these two are connected.

I wish you luck and happiness as you embark on the journey of treating hearing loss, restoring clarity, increasing independence, and keeping a healthy and fit brain!

EPILOGUE

You Had Questions and I hope I've Provided Answers

SO, THERE YOU HAVE IT! Twenty-one of my patents' most popular questions answered (for your convenience I've included a handy FAQ directly after this epilogue that summarizes most, if not all, of the questions we've just covered. Consider it a handy "quick reference" of sorts). The fact is no book can ever answer EVERY question for every patient. Every case is unique, just as every patient with hearing loss that I treat is different. What I've tried to do is provide you with the basics and hopefully the confidence you'll need to ask further questions of your own hearing health provider when the time comes.

This is your hearing, your brain, and your overall health we are talking about here; never be afraid to insist on being heard and having your questions answered by your clinician. Now that you're armed with the answers for today's most frequently asked audiology questions, you can finally make the right decision for you or a loved one when embarking on the journey of medical treatment for hearing loss.

To take the next step, schedule your hearing evaluation and consultation with an Audigy member-clinic.

FAQS

A RESOURCE GUIDE OF FREQUENTLY ASKED QUESTIONS & TERMINOLOGY

What might happen if I wait to treat my hearing loss?

Even mild hearing loss can be a major problem for a number of reasons. Hearing loss can increase the risk of developing dementia and is correlated with several other major diseases including diabetes, coronary disease, kidney disease, and increased risk of falling. Early treatment also improves the treatment prognosis and expected outcomes.

Who are some famous people who've invested in treating their hearing loss with technology?

The list is quite long! A (much) abbreviated list includes presidents Reagan, Clinton, and George H.W. Bush, and other celebrities and famous athletes including Huey Lewis, Lou Ferrigno, William Shatner, Pete Townshend, Whoopi Goldberg, Derrick Coleman, Congressman Jim Ryun, Phil Collins, and Brian Kerwin.

Will I be able to afford NeuroTechnology™?

Yes. Not only are hearing loss treatment options more affordable than ever, but insurance, payment plans, flexible spending accounts,, and a variety of other financing options make this an all but moot point.

Will being fit with NeuroTechnology™ be painful or obvious to others?

No and no. Advances in miniaturization of technology have helped develop the most light-weight, discrete, and sometimes completely invisible technology ever used to treat hearing loss.

Will I have to miss work or other social activities to be fit with NeuroTechnology™?

The initial comprehensive evaluation and treatment procedures will take between one to one and a half hours. Follow-up visits after that will only take between fifteen to thirty minutes. Patients walk out of the office after the first appointment and go about their lives...only now they can hear **MUCH** better!

Is it really such a big deal if I don't treat my hearing loss?

Yes. Too many people believe that their hearing loss is "normal for their age." There is no such thing as "normal" or "age-corrected" hearing loss. Hearing loss is a progressive degenerative disorder that will continue to negatively impact your life and cognition the longer it goes untreated.

What are some of the warning signs that I may have hearing loss?

Early symptoms of hearing loss include difficulty following conversation in background noise, experiencing tinnitus (ringing in the ears), having to turn up the TV louder than others need it, asking people to repeat often, finding yourself needing to read lips to hear better, difficulty understanding on the phone, and your family bugging you about getting help.

What kind of side-effects can result from NOT treating my hearing loss?

Untreated hearing loss is implicated in increased risk of falls, development of dementia, diabetes, coronary disease, depression, as well as increased stress and reduced physical activity.

Why should I choose a specialist to treat my hearing loss?

Hearing loss is a major medical condition and has been listed as the **third most common** medical disorder impacting seniors. Unfortunately, loopholes in many state and federal laws allow for traditional hearing aids to be sold online and in retail establishments, including some of the big-box discount stores. These traditional hearing aids are most often older models and are only designed to amplify sound.

NeuroTechnology™, designed to treat the cognitive aspects of hearing loss, is the "gold-standard" and considered "best practices" by audiologists and board-certified specialists in private practice audiology clinics.

How do I know if my hearing care provider is a doctor of audiology?

This is typically pretty easy to figure out by searching the internet or even calling the office. I've never been bothered by a patient calling to confirm my credentials prior to his or her arrival—in fact, I believe this shows a proper amount of due diligence on the part of the patient and a true investment in his or her hearing health care. Most states will also provide a list or search tool online to find licensed and certified providers.

What is a Patient Care Coordinator?

During your initial consultation(s), you will usually be assigned a patient contact person—we call this person a Patient Care Coordinator in our office—with whom to schedule appointments, confer with for rescheduling, and, of course, help you get answers to any and all questions you may have at any point in the process.

Why are follow-up visits important?

These are wonderful opportunities to ask questions you may have missed the first time, get further details from your specialist, and bring a family member to learn about your diagnosis and treatment plan.

Why is early treatment so important?

Since we recommend adults fifty and older to have a comprehensive hearing evaluation, we use the term "Ears and Rears"! This is meant to remind people to add hearing to their list of medical appointments once they turn fifty. At fifty, if the patient is found to have hearing loss, it is critical to start treatment early to avoid some of the devastating consequences of untreated hearing loss. Alternatively, if the patient has normal hearing, a baseline will be established and used for comparison at follow-up appointments.

What if I don't believe in early treatment of age-related hearing loss?

I can only emphasize that research into the auditory system supports early treatment. Talk to someone you trust about your concerns or reservations. Unfortunately, for many patients it takes nearly seven years for them to admit they have hearing loss (or to succumb to pressure from family members) and start treatment. By this time, the hearing loss will typically be at a moderate degree or beyond and, in some cases, treatment outcomes can be negatively impacted. To assure a positive prognosis and improved treatment outcomes, hearing loss must be caught early and treated early to maintain positive connections to the brain. *"Catch it early and treat it early!"*

What is sensorineural hearing loss?

Sensorineural hearing loss (SNHL) is a hearing impairment that results from damage to, or dysfunction of, the inner ear (cochlear) and/or the auditory nervous system. Age-related hearing loss is a form of sensorineural hearing loss.

What is a conductive hearing loss?

Conductive hearing loss (CHL) is a hearing impairment that results from damage to, or dysfunction of, the outer ear (pinna and ear canal) and/or the middle ear (the eardrum or ossicles—hammer, anvil, and stirrup). In some cases of CHL, medical or surgical intervention can help restore hearing function.

What is a processing disorder?

Hearing loss is often defined in terms of the amount of lost volume that results from either a SNHL or a CHL. However, many patients, even those with normal hearing levels, can have a processing disorder that will limit their ability to understand and follow speech in background noise. The noise cancellation feature in NeuroTechnology™ provides significant benefit by reducing background noise and enhancing speech—even for those with normal hearing.

Should I bring a family member with me to my appointment(s)?

I answer this with a decisive YES. Your hearing loss not only impacts you but also everybody around you. I have always encouraged every patient to bring a spouse or a loved one to every appointment so he or she can help me, and the patient, better understand the daily impact of hearing loss on everybody's life. It is also important to assess how your family member speaks. Are they a "soft talker" or do they really mumble? It also helps me to know more about how you communicate with each other.

What is NeuroTechnology™?

In recent years, traditional hearing aids, which simply make sounds louder, have been phased out and replaced with NeuroTechnology™. The significant cognitive benefits to NeuroTechnology™ include: **binaural processing** (two ears working together), **sound orientation** (ability to detect the source of incoming sounds with increased accuracy), **enhanced clarity of voices** (even soft speakers), automatic **adaptation to environment** (no more pushing buttons and adjusting volume), and **noise-cancellation** filtering of background noise to enhance hearing conversation in noisy environments (hearing better in crowded rooms, restaurants, etc.).

What is the primary benefit of NeuroTechnology™?

This answer is outlined in greater detail throughout the book. In summary, recent reports find that NeuroTechnology™ and the treatment of hearing loss can significantly improve quality of life, reduce the risk of developing dementia, and offer an increase in cognitive function. Yes, all of this can be achieved by treating your hearing loss.

How do I get started with NeuroTechnology™?

It's simple: Request an appointment with the local audiology clinic that sent you this book or visit **www.ExcellenceinAudiology.org** to find a member-clinic in your area. Your initial consultation/exam will most likely be covered by your insurance.

Is getting traditional hearing aids still effective treatment for hearing loss?

For the majority of patients, traditional hearing aids will not effectively treat hearing loss or the symptoms of hearing loss, including tinnitus. Traditional hearing aids are volume-enhancing devices that may help certain people in very limited environments (e.g., conversing one-on- one in a room with no background noise). For patients needing to follow conversation in dynamic environments (e.g., sitting at a dinner table with family and friends, going out to a restaurant, sitting in a lecture hall or a place of worship, playing cards with others, etc.), NeuroTechnology™ will restore clarity and enhance speech even in background noise.

What are some of my payment options besides insurance?

One way many patients pay for their NeuroTechnology™ is by utilizing Flexible Spending through their work insurance plan, financing at 0%or a fixed rate, or even taking advantage of the new financing program offered by many of the Audigy member-clinics.

What if I need an emergency appointment before or after office hours?

(This answer is a bit longer than most because of the seriousness of some audiology emergencies) Audiology emergencies most often fall in to one of two categories:

Sudden Change in Hearing

While rare, a sudden change in hearing can occur. This medical condition, known as sudden-onset sensorineural hearing loss, may occur in one, or both (even more rare), ears and is often associated with a virus (and sometimes occurs in tandem with an upper respiratory infection). There is varying data on successful treatment protocols for this disorder; regardless, the key to potentially recovering hearing function requires seeking medical attention within 24-48 hours of initial symptoms. If you suspect you have a sudden hearing loss, contact your audiologist or primary care physician for immediate assistance.

Emergency Related to the NeuroTechnology™

Broken or "non-functioning devices" may occur from time to time during your treatment. If there is any disturbance, such as lost domes, tight speaker wires, or irritation, call your hearing care provider's office as soon as possible to have them evaluate the urgency of the problem and schedule you to be seen accordingly. Most offices will have special emergency appointments set aside each day to help in these situations.

In the interim, here are helpful hints to remedy some of the problems that you may encounter until you can be seen in the office:

- Itching is normal in the early stages of wearing devices. It is important to be sure your dome or earmold is clean.
- A device causing feedback or "squealing" can generally be worn until you are seen by our team. Call the office as soon as you notice this feedback or squealing so that we can schedule you to make a prescription change.
- A dome, earmold, or removable device that is not fitting well is not to be worn until it can be properly adjusted at the office. Call the office as soon as possible to have your specialists make the adjustment for comfort and fit.

Can NeuroTechnology™ get wet?

Unlike traditional hearing aids that had no moisture resistance, most of today's NeuroTechnology™ comes with an IP57 rating for dust and moisture resistance. In lay terms, the "IP" stands for International Protection Rating and the "5" indicates the unit is dust protected (highest score is a 6 on this scale) and the "7" indicates the unit can be immersed in up to one meter of water (that is over three feet!). With that said—we continue to direct patients to not swim or bathe with their NeuroTechnology™.

Should I sleep with my NeuroTechnology™?

It is recommended to not sleep with your NeuroTechnology™ for three reasons:

- Sleeping with the device on can cause discomfort to the ear and side of the head. Give your ears a rest.
- It is easier for a device to fall out when you turn over in bed and may get lost.

- Your batteries will wear out more quickly. If using disposable batteries, you will have to change them every few days. If your devices are rechargeable, you will have to remove them and recharge them during waking hours (takes about 3-5 hours).

However, I do have patients that sleep with their NeuroTechnology™ for safety and personal reasons.

How do I regularly clean my NeuroTechnology™?

Like with cleaning your home…clean it a little each day and it won't become such a mess! Your audiologist will help you understand daily and monthly routines for maintaining your NeuroTechnology™ at home. Use a lint free cloth and brush (typically provided at your first treatment appointment) to wipe down the unit every day. This will help prevent oils from the skin, dandruff, earwax, and other environmental dust from clogging the microphones and speaker over time. I also encourage my patients to change the "parts" as needed (this could be once a month or every few months depending on your issues). This includes wax filters (designed to prevent earwax from entering the unit), domes (designed to securely hold the unit in the ear) and different microphone filters (included on some NeuroTechnology™ options).

BIBLIOGRAPHY

THE SCIENCE BEHIND EVERYTHING YOU READ IN THIS BOOK

If you read this book, chances are that you or a family member are struggling to deal with the impact of hearing loss on your social, physical, and mental well-being. By now, I hope that you have come to understand the negative impact of untreated hearing loss on overall quality of life and cognitive function. I thank you for taking your hearing healthcare seriously and for allowing me to provide the education necessary for you to make an informed decision about medically treating your hearing loss.

Hear Better, Live Better,
Dr. Jewell (aka the EarNerd)

Audiology and Hearing Health
3050 Business Park Circle, Suite 303
Goodlettsville, TN 37072
(615) 448-6745
www.audiologyandhearing.com

This book is the result of my 39+ years in hearing health care. In this time, I have amassed information from my research, reading of scientific publications, in professional meetings (as the listener and the presenter), and from directly interacting with patients' and their loved ones. Below is a list of references that helped me put together this book and present the information to you in a succinct manner. You can access these manuscripts on Google Scholar and/or Pubmed.

"Active Ageing: A Policy Framework." *The Aging Male* 5, no. 1 (2002), 1-37.

Adult Cognition and Hearing Aids. U of Canterbury. Communication Disorders, 2015.

Agmon, Maayan, Limor Lavie, and Michail Doumas. "The Association between Hearing Loss, Postural Control, and Mobility in Older Adults: A Systematic Review." *Journal of the American Academy of Audiology* 28, no. 6 (2017), 575-588.

"Association of Hearing Impairment and Subsequent Driving Mobility in Older Adults." *The Gerontologist* 55, no. Suppl_2 (2015), 137-138.

Bainbridge, Kathleen E., Howard J. Hoffman, and Catherine C. Cowie. "Diabetes and Hearing Impairment in the United States: Audiometric Evidence from the National Health and Nutrition Examination Survey, 1999 to 2004." *Annals of Internal Medicine* 149, no. 1 (2008), 1.

Bassuk, Shari S., Thomas A. Glass, and Lisa F. Berkman. "Social Disengagement and Incident Cognitive Decline in Community-Dwelling Elderly Persons." *Annals of Internal Medicine* 131, no. 3 (1999), 165.

Bernabei, Roberto, Ubaldo Bonuccelli, Stefania Maggi, Alessandra Marengoni, Alessandro Martini, Maurizio Memo, Sergio Pecorelli, Andrea P. Peracino, Nicola Quaranta, and Roberto Stella. "Hearing loss and cognitive decline in older adults: questions and answers." *Aging Clinical and Experimental Research* 26, no. 6 (2014), 567-573.

Burns, Elizabeth R., Judy A. Stevens, and Robin Lee. "The direct costs of fatal and non-fatal falls among older adults — United States." *Journal of Safety Research* 58 (2016), 99-103.

Cardin, Velia. "Effects of Aging and Adult-Onset Hearing Loss on Cortical Auditory Regions." *Frontiers in Neuroscience* 10 (2016).

Cass, SP. "Alzheimer's Disease and Exercise: A Literature Review." *Curr. Sports Med. Rep*, February 16, 2017.

Chen, David S., Dane J. Genther, Joshua Betz, and Frank R. Lin. "Association Between Hearing Impairment and Self-Reported Difficulty in Physical Functioning." *Journal of the American Geriatrics Society* 62, no. 5 (2014), 850-856.

Chia, Ee-Munn, Jie J. Wang, Elena Rochtchina, Robert R. Cumming, Philip Newall, and Paul Mitchell. "Hearing Impairment and Health-Related Quality of Life: The Blue Mountains Hearing Study." *Ear and Hearing* 28, no. 2 (2007), 187-195.

Collins, John G. "Prevalence of Selected Chronic Conditions: United States, 1983-85." *PsycEXTRA Dataset* (n.d.).

Davidson, JGS. "Older Adults With a Combination of Vision and Hearing Impairment Experience Higher Rates of Cognitive Impairment, Functional Dependence, and Worse Outcomes Across a Set of Quality Indicators." Last modified August 1, 2017.

De Leon, M. J., S. DeSanti, R. Zinkowski, P. D. Mehta, D. Pratico, S. Segal, C. Clark, D. Kerkman, J. DeBernardis, and J. Li. "MRI and CSF studies in the early diagnosis of Alzheimer's disease." *Journal of Internal Medicine* 256, no. 3 (2004), 205-223.

Deal, Jennifer A., Josh Betz, Kristine Yaffe, Tamara Harris, Elizabeth Purchase-Helzner, Suzanne Satterfield, Sheila Pratt, Nandini Govil, Eleanor M. Simonsick, and Frank R. Lin. "Hearing Impairment and Incident Dementia and Cognitive Decline in Older Adults: The Health ABC Study." *The Journals of Gerontology Series A: Biological Sciences and Medical Sciences*, 2016, glw069.

"Dementia Prevention, Intervention, and Care." *Lancet*, July 19, 2017.

Desjardins, Jamie L. "Analysis of Performance on Cognitive Test Measures Before, During, and After 6 Months of Hearing Aid Use: A Single-Subject Experimental Design." *American Journal of Audiology* 25, no. 2 (2016), 127.

Ferreira, Lidiane M., Alberto N. Ramos, and Eveline P. Mendes. "Characterization of tinnitus in the elderly and its possible related disorders." *Brazilian Journal of Otorhinolaryngology*75, no. 2 (2009), 249-255.

Genther, Dane J., Joshua Betz, Sheila Pratt, Kathryn R. Martin, Tamara B. Harris, Suzanne Satterfield, Douglas C. Bauer, Anne B. Newman, Eleanor M. Simonsick, and Frank R. Lin. "Association Between Hearing Impairment and Risk of Hospitalization in Older Adults." *Journal of the American Geriatrics Society* 63, no. 6 (2015), 1146-1152.

Gibrin, PC, AN Ramos Junior, and EP Mendes. "Prevalence of Tinnitus Complaints and Probable Association with Hearing Loss, Diabetes Mellitus and Hypertension in Elderly." *Codas*, 2013.

Gispen, Fiona E., David S. Chen, Dane J. Genther, and Frank R. Lin. "Association

Between Hearing Impairment and Lower Levels of Physical Activity in Older Adults." *Journal of the American Geriatrics Society* 62, no. 8 (2014), 1427-1433.

Govender, SM, CD Govender, and G. Matthews. "Cochlear Function in Patients with Chronic Kidney Disease." *South African/Commun Diord*, December 2013.

Haan, Mary N. "Can Social Engagement Prevent Cognitive Decline in Old Age?" *Annals of Internal Medicine* 131, no. 3 (1999), 220.

"Hearing Impairment and Frailty in English Community-Dwelling Older Adults: A 4-Year Follow-Up Study." *The Gerontologist* 56, no. Suppl_3 (2016), 319-319.

"Hearing Loss and Cognitive Decline in Older Adults." *JAMA Internal Medicine*, February 25, 2013.

"The Impact of Hearing Loss on Quality of Life in Older Adults." *Gerontologist*, October 2003.

"The Impact of Hearing Loss on quality of Life in Older Adults." *Gerontologist*, October 2003.

"An Introduction to MarkeTrak IX: A New Baseline for the Hearing Aid Market." *Hearing Review*, May 15, 2015.

Jacoby, R., and R. Levy. "CT Scanning and the Investigation of Dementia: A Review." *J.R. Soc. Med*, May 1980.

Jamaldeen, Jishana, Aneesh Basheer, Akhil Sarma, and Ravichandran Kandasamy. "Prevalence and patterns of hearing loss among chronic kidney disease patients undergoing haemodialysis." *australasian medical journal*, 2015, 41-46.

Kamil, Rebecca J., Lingsheng Li, and Frank R. Lin. "Association between Hearing Impairment and Frailty in Older Adults." *Journal of the American Geriatrics Society* 62, no. 6 (2014), 1186-1188.

Kelley, Amy S., Kathleen McGarry, Rebecca Gorges, and Jonathan S. Skinner. "The Burden of Health Care Costs for Patients With Dementia in the Last 5 Years of Life." *Annals of Internal Medicine* 163, no. 10 (2015), 729.

Kochkin, Sergei. "MarkeTrak VII." *The Hearing Journal* 60, no. 4 (2007), 24-51.

Lambert, Justin, Rouzbeh Ghadry-Tavi, Kate Knuff, Marc Jutras, Jodi Siever, Paul Mick, Carolyn Roque, Gareth Jones, Jonathan Little, and Harry Miller. "Targeting functional fitness, hearing and health-related quality of life in older adults with hearing loss: Walk, Talk 'n' Listen, study protocol for a pilot randomized controlled trial." *Trials* 18, no. 1 (2017).

Le Goff, Nicolas, Dorothea Wendt, Thomas Lunner, and Elaine Ng. "Opn Clinical Evidence. Oticon White Paper." 2016.

Lin, F.R., L. Ferrucci, Y. An, J.O. Goh, Jimit Doshi, E.J. Metter, C. Davatzikos, M.A. Kraut, and S.M. Resnick. "Association of hearing impairment with brain volume changes in older adults." *NeuroImage* 90 (2014), 84-92.

Lin, Frank R. "Hearing Loss Prevalence in the United States." *Archives of Internal Medicine*171, no. 20 (2011), 1851.

Lin, Frank R. "Hearing Loss and Falls Among Older Adults in the United States." *Archives of Internal Medicine* 172, no. 4 (2012), 369.

Lin, Frank R., E. J. Metter, Richard J. O'Brien, Susan M. Resnick, Alan B. Zonderman, and Luigi Ferrucci. "Hearing Loss and Incident Dementia." *Archives of Neurology* 68, no. 2 (2011).

Martini, Alessandro, Alessandro Castiglione, Roberto Bovo, Antonino Vallesi, and Carlo Gabelli. "Aging, Cognitive Load, Dementia and Hearing Loss." *Audiology and Neurotology* 19, no. 1 (2014), 2-5.

Meister, Hartmut, Stefan Schreitmüller, Magdalene Ortmann, Sebastian Rählmann, and Martin Walger. "Effects of Hearing Loss and Cognitive Load on Speech Recognition with Competing Talkers." *Frontiers in Psychology* 7 (2016).

Melse-Boonstra, Alida, and Ian Mackenzie. "Iodine deficiency, thyroid function and hearing deficit: a review." *Nutrition Research Reviews* 26, no. 02 (2013), 110-117.

Meyerhoff, William L. "The Thyroid and Audition." *The Laryngoscope* 86, no. 4 (1976), 483-489.

Miyawaki, Christina E., E. D. Bouldin, G. S. Kumar, and L. C. McGuire. "Associations between physical activity and cognitive functioning among middle-aged and older adults." *The journal of nutrition, health & aging* 21, no. 6 (2016), 637-647.

Mulrow, Cynthia D., Christine Aguilar, James E. Endicott, Ramon Velez, Michael R. Tuley, Walter S. Charlip, and Judith A. Hill. "Association Between Hearing Impairment and the Quality of Life of Elderly Individuals." *Journal of the American Geriatrics Society* 38, no. 1 (1990), 45-50.

Oh, Esther, Frank Lin, and Sara Mamo. "Enhancing Communication in Adults with Dementia and Age-Related Hearing Loss." *Seminars in Hearing* 38, no. 02 (2017), 177-183.

Palmer, Andrew D., Jason T. Newsom, and Karen S. Rook. "How does difficulty communicating affect the social relationships of older adults? An exploration using data from a national survey." *Journal of Communication Disorders* 62 (2016), 131-146.

Popelka, Michael M., Karen J. Cruickshanks, Terry L. Wiley, Theodore S. Tweed, Barbara E. Klein, and Ronald Klein. "Low Prevalence of Hearing Aid Use Among Older Adults with Hearing Loss: The Epidemiology of Hearing Loss Study." *Journal of the American Geriatrics Society* 46, no. 9 (1998), 1075-1078.

Qian, Z. J., Peter D. Chang, Gul Moonis, and Anil K. Lalwani. "A novel method of quantifying brain atrophy associated with age-related hearing loss." *NeuroImage: Clinical* 16 (2017), 205-209.

Qian, Zhen J., Kapil Wattamwar, Francesco F. Caruana, Jenna Otter, Matthew J. Leskowitz, Barbara Siedlecki, Jaclyn B. Spitzer, and Anil K. Lalwani. "Hearing Aid Use is Associated with Better Mini-Mental State Exam Performance." *The American Journal of Geriatric Psychiatry* 24, no. 9 (2016), 694-702.

Ryu, Nam-Gyu, Il J. Moon, Hayoung Byun, Sun H. Jin, Heesung Park, Kyu-Sun Jang, and Yang-Sun Cho. "Clinical effectiveness of wireless CROS (contralateral routing of offside signals) hearing aids." *European Archives of Oto-Rhino-Laryngology* 272, no. 9 (2014), 2213-2219.

Seimetz, Bruna, Adriane Teixeira, Leticia Rosito, Leticia Flores, Carlos Pappen, and Celso Dall'igna. "Pitch and Loudness Tinnitus in Individuals with Presbycusis." *International Archives of Otorhinolaryngology* 20, no. 04 (2016), 321-326.

Sindhusake, Doungkamol, Paul Mitchell, Philip Newall, Maryanne Golding, Elena Rochtchina, and George Rubin. "Prevalence and characteristics of tinnitus in older adults: the Blue Mountains Hearing Study: Prevalencia y características del acúfeno en adultos mayores: el Estudio de Audición Blue Mountains." *International Journal of Audiology* 42, no. 5 (2003), 289-294.

Snapp, Hillary A., Fred D. Holt, Xuezhong Liu, and Suhrud M. Rajguru. "Comparison of Speech-in-Noise and Localization Benefits in Unilateral Hearing Loss Subjects Using Contralateral Routing of Signal Hearing Aids or Bone-Anchored Implants." *Otology & Neurotology* 38, no. 1 (2017), 11-18.

"Social Isolation in Community-Dwelling Seniors: An Evidence-Based Analysis." *Health Quality Ontario*, August 2008.

Spulber, Gabriela, Eini Niskanen, Stuart MacDonald, Oded Smilovici, Kewei Chen, Eric M. Reiman, Anne M. Jauhiainen, Merja Hallikainen, Susanna Tervo, and Lars-Olof Wahlund. "Whole brain atrophy rate predicts progression from MCI to Alzheimer's disease." *Neurobiology of Aging* 31, no. 9 (2010), 1601-1605.

Su, Peijen, Chih-Chao Hsu, Hung-Ching Lin, Wei-Shin Huang, Tsung-Lin Yang, Wei-Ting Hsu, Cheng-Li Lin, Chung-Yi Hsu, Kuang-Hsi Chang, and Yi-Chao Hsu. "Age-related hearing loss and dementia: a 10-year national population-based study." *European Archives of Oto-Rhino-Laryngology* 274, no. 5 (2017), 2327-2334.

Vignesh, S. S., V. Jaya, Anand Moses, and A. Muraleedharan. "Identifying Early Onset of Hearing Loss in Young Adults With Diabetes Mellitus Type 2 Using High Frequency Audiometry." *Indian Journal of Otolaryngology and Head & Neck Surgery* 67, no. 3 (2014), 234-237.

Weinstein, Barbara E. *Hearing Impairment and Social Isolation in the Elderly*. publisher not identified, 1980.

Yates, J.A., L. Clare, and B. Woods. "You've Got a Friend in Me: Can Social Engagement Mediate the Relationship Between Mood and MCI?" *Innovation in Aging* 1, no. suppl_1 (2017), 1179-1179.

Yates, Jennifer A., Linda Clare, and Robert T. Woods. "What is the Relationship between Health, Mood, and Mild Cognitive Impairment?" *Journal of Alzheimer's Disease* 55, no. 3 (2016), 1183-1193.

Zheng, Yuqiu, Shengnuo Fan, Wang Liao, Wenli Fang, Songhua Xiao, and Jun Liu. "Hearing impairment and risk of Alzheimer's disease: a meta-analysis of prospective cohort studies." *Neurological Sciences* 38, no. 2 (2016), 233-239.

www.ingramcontent.com/pod-product-compliance
Lightning Source LLC
LaVergne TN
LVHW021141160826
845679LV00023B/2002

* 9 7 9 8 8 6 8 9 3 1 6 1 1 *